AF901826

Methods in Molecular Biology

Series Editor
John M. Walker
School of Life and Medical Sciences
University of Hertfordshire
Hatfield, Hertfordshire, UK

For further volumes:
http://www.springer.com/series/7651

For over 35 years, biological scientists have come to rely on the research protocols and methodologies in the critically acclaimed *Methods in Molecular Biology* series. The series was the first to introduce the step-by-step protocols approach that has become the standard in all biomedical protocol publishing. Each protocol is provided in readily-reproducible step-by-step fashion, opening with an introductory overview, a list of the materials and reagents needed to complete the experiment, and followed by a detailed procedure that is supported with a helpful notes section offering tips and tricks of the trade as well as troubleshooting advice. These hallmark features were introduced by series editor Dr. John Walker and constitute the key ingredient in each and every volume of the *Methods in Molecular Biology* series. Tested and trusted, comprehensive and reliable, all protocols from the series are indexed in PubMed.

Mouse Models of Cancer

Methods and Protocols

Edited by

Maja Čemažar, Tanja Jesenko and Urša Lampreht Tratar

Institute of Oncology Ljubljana, Ljubljana, Slovenia

Humana Press

Editors
Maja Čemažar
Institute of Oncology Ljubljana
Ljubljana, Slovenia

Tanja Jesenko
Institute of Oncology Ljubljana
Ljubljana, Slovenia

Urša Lampreht Tratar
Institute of Oncology Ljubljana
Ljubljana, Slovenia

ISSN 1064-3745 ISSN 1940-6029 (electronic)
Methods in Molecular Biology
ISBN 978-1-0716-3713-5 ISBN 978-1-0716-3714-2 (eBook)
https://doi.org/10.1007/978-1-0716-3714-2

© The Editor(s) (if applicable) and The Author(s), under exclusive license to Springer Science+Business Media, LLC, part of Springer Nature 2024
This work is subject to copyright. All rights are solely and exclusively licensed by the Publisher, whether the whole or part of the material is concerned, specifically the rights of translation, reprinting, reuse of illustrations, recitation, broadcasting, reproduction on microfilms or in any other physical way, and transmission or information storage and retrieval, electronic adaptation, computer software, or by similar or dissimilar methodology now known or hereafter developed.
The use of general descriptive names, registered names, trademarks, service marks, etc. in this publication does not imply, even in the absence of a specific statement, that such names are exempt from the relevant protective laws and regulations and therefore free for general use.
The publisher, the authors, and the editors are safe to assume that the advice and information in this book are believed to be true and accurate at the date of publication. Neither the publisher nor the authors or the editors give a warranty, expressed or implied, with respect to the material contained herein or for any errors or omissions that may have been made. The publisher remains neutral with regard to jurisdictional claims in published maps and institutional affiliations.

This Humana imprint is published by the registered company Springer Science+Business Media, LLC, part of Springer Nature.
The registered company address is: 1 New York Plaza, New York, NY 10004, U.S.A.

Paper in this product is recyclable.

Preface

It all started in the early 1900s in the USA, in Massachusetts. It was the beginning of the modern era of using mice in scientific research, first for genetic studies, but soon after also for cancer studies, especially after the creation of the first inbred mouse, the C57Bl/6, developed by Clarence Cook Little.

Thereafter, the use of mouse models increased steadily, as mice and humans share about 70% of the same protein-coding gene sequences. Mouse models play a crucial role in cancer research as they provide a controlled and reproducible experimental system to study different aspects of cancer biology, including prevention, development, progression, and treatment, all of which are studied at different levels: the microenvironment, the mezzo-environment (organ level), and the macro-environment (whole organism). These models, which are often genetically modified or implanted with human tumor cells, offer insights into cancer development that are difficult to gain through clinical trials alone.

The development of the use of mouse models in cancer research has been further advanced by the application of the 3R (Replacement, Reduction, and Refinement) principles. The application of the 3R principles in cancer mouse model research helps to ensure that research is conducted ethically and minimizes the use of animals while maintaining scientific rigor. In addition, the implementation of ARRIVE (Animal Research Reporting In Vivo Experiments) and PREPARE (Planning Research and Experimental Procedures on Animals: Recommendations for Excellence) guidelines in mouse cancer research has improved the quality and translational value of the research.

Mouse models are an irreplaceable tool for understanding tumor development and progression by investigating how specific mutations contribute to the development and progression of cancer. Mouse cancer models are used to test potential cancer therapies, including chemotherapy, targeted therapies, and immunotherapies. The efficacy, toxicity, and safety of different treatments can be evaluated to identify promising candidates for further testing in clinical trials. In addition, mouse models can be used to study the mechanisms underlying treatment resistance so that strategies can be developed to overcome it. Mouse models are also suitable for the study of personalized medicine. In patient-derived xenograft models, human tumor tissue is implanted into mice. These models allow researchers to test a patient's specific tumor response to different therapies, facilitating personalized treatment approaches. In addition, mouse models can also be used to study the effects of lifestyle factors, environmental influences, and preventive measures on cancer development, contributing to the development of cancer prevention strategies.

This book presents various models for cancer studies, from leukemia and lymphoma models to different types of subcutaneous and orthotopic models. In addition, models for the healing process and the assessment of the immune response after local ablative therapies are discussed. The final chapters of the book deal with different imaging techniques that allow visualization of cancer at the cellular and tissue levels. Finally, a detailed description of necropsy is explained, which is essential for obtaining good biomaterial for translational research.

Ljubljana, Slovenia *Maja Čemažar*
Ljubljana, Slovenia *Tanja Jesenko*
Ljubljana, Slovenia *Urša Lamprebt Tratar*

Contents

Contributors

MAJA ANTOLIĆ • *Selvita, Zagreb, Croatia*
ELISABETH BELLARD • *Institut de Pharmacologie et de Biologie Structurale (IPBS), Université de Toulouse, CNRS, Université Toulouse III – Paul Sabatier (UT3), Toulouse, France*
LAURA BELVER • *Josep Carreras Leukemia Research Institute (IJC), Barcelona, Catalonia, Spain; Catalan Institute of Oncology (ICO) – Immuno Procure, Barcelona, Catalonia, Spain*
TANJA BLAGUS • *Department of Experimental Oncology, Institute of Oncology Ljubljana, Ljubljana, Slovenia; Institute of Biochemistry and Molecular Genetics, Faculty of Medicine, University of Ljubljana, Ljubljana, Slovenia*
TIM BOZIC • *Department of Experimental Oncology, Institute of Oncology Ljubljana, Ljubljana, Slovenia*
ANNA CAMPAGNARI • *Josep Carreras Leukemia Research Institute (IJC), Barcelona, Catalonia, Spain; Catalan Institute of Oncology (ICO) – Immuno Procure, Barcelona, Catalonia, Spain*
MAJA ČEMAŽAR • *Department of Experimental Oncology, Institute of Oncology Ljubljana, Ljubljana, Slovenia; Faculty of Health Sciences, University of Primorska, Isola, Slovenia*
SNJEŽANA ČUŽIĆ • *Selvita, Zagreb, Croatia*
MARIANGELA DE ROBERTIS • *Department of Biosciences, Biotechnology and Environment, University of Bari 'A. Moro', Bari, Italy*
LEO EDLINGER • *Division of Oncology, Department of Internal Medicine, Medical University of Graz, Graz, Austria*
ANDREJA ERMAN • *Faculty of Medicine, Institute of Cell Biology, Ljubljana, Slovenia*
ANJA GOLOB-URBANC • *Department of Synthetic Biology and Immunology, National Institute of Chemistry, Ljubljana, Slovenia*
MURIEL GOLZIO • *Institut de Pharmacologie et de Biologie Structurale (IPBS), Université de Toulouse, CNRS, Université Toulouse III – Paul Sabatier (UT3), Toulouse, France*
TANJA JESENKO • *Department of Experimental Oncology, Institute of Oncology Ljubljana, Ljubljana, Slovenia; Faculty of Medicine, University of Ljubljana, Ljubljana, Slovenia*
URŠKA KAMENŠEK • *Department of Experimental Oncology, Institute of Oncology, Ljubljana, Slovenia; Biotechnical Faculty, University of Ljubljana, Ljubljana, Slovenia*
TILEN KOMEL • *Department of Experimental Oncology, Institute of Oncology Ljubljana, Ljubljana, Slovenia*
ŠPELA KOS • *Department of Experimental Oncology, Institute of Oncology Ljubljana, Ljubljana, Slovenia*
ANDREJA KOZAK • *Department of Biochemistry and Molecular and Structural Biology, Jozef Stefan Institute, Ljubljana, Slovenia*
SIMONA KRANJC BREZAR • *Department of Experimental Oncology, Institute of Oncology, Ljubljana, Slovenia*
DUŠKO LAINŠČEK • *Department of Synthetic Biology and Immunology, National Institute of Chemistry, Ljubljana, Slovenia; EN-FIST Centre of Excellence, Ljubljana, Slovenia*
URŠA LAMPREHT TRATAR • *Veterinary Faculty, University of Ljubljana, Ljubljana, Slovenia; Department of Experimental Oncology, Institute of Oncology Ljubljana, Ljubljana, Slovenia*

BOSTJAN MARKELC • *Department of Experimental Oncology, Institute of Oncology Ljubljana, Ljubljana, Slovenia*
GEORGY MIKHAYLOV • *Department of Biochemistry and Molecular and Structural Biology, Jozef Stefan Institute, Ljubljana, Slovenia; SwissLumix SARL, Lausanne, Switzerland*
VUK MILUTINOVIĆ • *Selvita, Zagreb, Croatia*
ZIVA MODIC • *Department of Experimental Oncology, Institute of Oncology Ljubljana, Ljubljana, Slovenia; Faculty of Medicine, University of Ljubljana, Ljubljana, Slovenia*
ANJA OGNJENOVIĆ • *Selvita, Zagreb, Croatia*
SARA OREHEK • *Department of Synthetic Biology and Immunology, National Institute of Chemistry, Ljubljana, Slovenia; Graduate School of Biomedicine, University of Ljubljana, Ljubljana, Slovenia*
DOMINIKA PESKAR • *Faculty of Medicine, Institute of Cell Biology, Ljubljana, Slovenia*
TINKARA REMIC • *Institute of Pathology, Faculty of Medicine, University of Ljubljana, Ljubljana, Slovenia*
MARIANGELA DE ROBERTIS • *Department of Biosciences, Biotechnology and Biopharmaceutics, University of Bari 'A. Moro', Bari, Italy*
ROK ROMIH • *Faculty of Medicine, Institute of Cell Biology, University of Ljubljana, Ljubljana, Slovenia*
GREGOR SERŠA • *Department of Experimental Oncology, Institute of Oncology Ljubljana, Ljubljana, Slovenia; Faculty of Health Sciences, University of Ljubljana, Ljubljana, Slovenia*
EMANUELA SIGNORI • *Laboratory of Molecular Pathology and Experimental Oncology, Institute of Translational Pharmacology, Consiglio Nazionale delle Ricerche, Rome, Italy*
KATJA URŠIČ VALENTINUZZI • *Department of Experimental Oncology, Institute of Oncology Ljubljana, Ljubljana, Slovenia; Biotechnical Faculty, University of Ljubljana, Ljubljana, Slovenia*
OLGA VASILJEVA • *Department of Biochemistry and Molecular and Structural Biology, Jozef Stefan Institute, Ljubljana, Slovenia; The Jozef Stefan International Postgraduate School, Ljubljana, Slovenia; OV: CytomX Therapeutics, Inc., South San Francisco, CA, USA*
PETER VERANIČ • *Faculty of Medicine, Institute of Cell Biology, Ljubljana, Slovenia*
DAŠA ZUPANČIČ • *Faculty of Medicine, Institute of Cell Biology, University of Ljubljana, Ljubljana, Slovenia*

Chapter 1

In Vivo Modeling of Leukemia by Murine Stem Cell Transplantation

Leo Edlinger

Abstract

Murine stem cell transplantation is a well-established method for the in vivo study of leukemic pathophysiology. Adoptive transfer of murine leukemic cells into lethally irradiated recipient mice leads to reconstitution of the hematopoietic system with malignant cells and eventually to leukemic progression in the recipient mice. Here, we describe the detailed protocol of the production of retroviral particles carrying the leukemic oncogene of interest as well as the isolation, retroviral transduction, and adoptive transfer of murine bone marrow cells.

Key words Leukemia, Mouse model, Hematopoietic stem cells, Stem cell transplantation, Retroviral transduction

1 Introduction

Various methods have been developed to mimic leukemic pathophysiology in vivo. These include carcinogen-induced (chemicals, irradiation, and viral infection) murine models, transgenic mouse models, adoptive transfer of murine hematopoietic cells (murine stem cell transplantation) into recipient mice, and xenograft models [1]. Here, we will focus on the murine stem cell transplantation to model leukemia in vivo.

Long-term hematopoietic stem cells (LT-HSCs) are required for the reconstitution of the host hematopoietic system [2]. Therefore, donor mice are treated with 5-fluorouracil (5-FU) to stimulate the proliferation of hematopoietic stem cells (HSCs) [2]. Meanwhile, replication-incompetent retroviral particles containing the leukemic oncogene of interest (e.g., *FLT3-ITD* or *BCR-ABL*) are produced in packaging cells [3]. HSC-enriched bone marrow of donor mice is isolated, cultured, and transduced with the oncogene-carrying retrovirus to induce leukemic transformation of HSCs. The cultured bone marrow cells are then

Maja Čemažar, Tanja Jesenko and Urša Lampreht Tratar (eds.), *Mouse Models of Cancer: Methods and Protocols*, Methods in Molecular Biology, vol. 2773, https://doi.org/10.1007/978-1-0716-3714-2_1,
© The Author(s), under exclusive license to Springer Science+Business Media, LLC, part of Springer Nature 2024

intravenously injected into lethally irradiated recipient mice. Hematopoietic reconstitution with malignant cells is followed by leukemic progression. Mice exhibiting severe symptoms of leukemia are euthanized and their organs can be used for further analysis. Alternatively, leukemic mice can be treated with cancer therapeutics and used for studying new treatment regimens.

2 Materials

2.1 Stimulation of HSC Proliferation in Donor Mice

1. 1 mL syringes and 26 G needles.
2. 10 mg/mL 5-FU diluted in phosphate-buffered saline (PBS).
3. 4–6-week-old isogenic donor mice for isolation of bone marrow cells.

2.2 Production of Retroviral Particles

1. Dulbecco's Modified Eagle's Medium (DMEM) containing 10% fetal calf serum (FCS), 1% penicillin/streptomycin, and 2 mM L-glutamine.
2. Phoenix ecotropic (Phoenix E) cells for production of retroviral particles (*see* **Note 1**).
3. 10 cm tissue culture dishes.
4. Retrovirus carrying the leukemic oncogene of interest (20 μg per 10 cm tissue culture dish of Phoenix E cells) (*see* **Note 2**).
5. Light microscope for estimation of confluency of Phoenix E cells.
6. Polystyrene tubes for calcium phosphate precipitation.
7. 0.25 M $CaCl_2$ solution and 0.22 μm filter.
8. 2× HBS buffer: 280 mM NaCl, 50 mM Hepes, 1.5 mM Na_2HPO_4, pH 6.95, and 0.22 μm filter.
9. 50 mM chloroquine.
10. Roswell Park Memorial Institute 1640 (RPMI 1640) medium containing 20% FCS, 1% penicillin/streptomycin, and 2 mM L-glutamine.
11. Fluorescence microscope for estimation of transfection efficiency.
12. 10 mL syringes and 0.45 μm filters.

2.3 Isolation of Bone Marrow Cells

1. RPMI 1640 medium containing 10% FCS, 1% penicillin/streptomycin, and 2 mM L-glutamine.
2. 5 mL syringes, 22 G needles, 40 μm cell strainers, and 15 mL conical tubes.
3. Red blood cell lysis buffer.
4. Hemocytometer for cell number determination.

5. 10 ng/mL recombinant murine interleukin 3 (IL 3), 10 ng/mL recombinant murine interleukin 6 (IL 6), and 100 ng/mL recombinant murine stem cell factor (SCF) (*see* **Note 3**).
6. RPMI 1640 medium containing 20% FCS, 1% penicillin/streptomycin, 2 mM L-glutamine, 10 ng/mL recombinant murine IL 3, 10 ng/mL recombinant murine IL 6, and 100 ng/mL recombinant murine SCF.
7. 12-well cell culture plates.

2.4 Transduction of Bone Marrow Cells

1. 10 ng/mL recombinant murine IL 3, 10 ng/mL recombinant murine IL 6, and 100 ng/mL recombinant murine SCF (*see* **Note 3**).
2. 10 mg/mL polybrene.

2.5 Stem Cell Transplantation

1. PBS.
2. Hemocytometer for cell number determination.
3. Flow cytometer for determination of transduction efficiency.
4. X-ray or γ-ray radiation source for lethal whole-body irradiation (9 Gy) of recipient mice – use an irradiation box for the mice.
5. 6–8-week-old isogenic recipient mice for murine stem cell transplantation.
6. 1 mL syringes, 26 G needles, and a mouse restrainer for intravenous injection.

2.6 Analysis

1. Automated veterinary analyzer for assessing blood differential cell count.
2. Flow cytometer to determine the number of fluorescently labeled leukemic cells.

3 Methods

3.1 Stimulation of HSC Proliferation in Donor Mice

Day -7: Intraperitoneal (i.p.) injection of 150 mg/kg 5-FU per isogenic donor mouse (4–6 weeks old) for induction of HSC proliferation [2].

3.2 Production of Retroviral Particles

Day -5: Seed 3×10^6 Phoenix E cells in 10 mL DMEM medium (containing 10% FCS, 1% penicillin/streptomycin, and 2 mM L-glutamine) in a 10 cm tissue culture dish.

Day -4: Retrovirally transfect Phoenix E cells at 70–80% confluency (*see* **Note 4**) with the leukemic oncogene of interest via the calcium phosphate-mediated transfection method [3]. For a 10 cm tissue culture dish of Phoenix E cells, use 20 μg of retroviral particles carrying the leukemic oncogene of interest. Prepare the calcium phosphate precipitation mix in a polystyrene tube. Filter the prepared 0.25 M $CaCl_2$ solution through a 0.22 μm filter. Add 1 mL of 0.25 M $CaCl_2$ to 20 μg of the retroviral particles. Filter the prepared 2× HBS buffer through a 0.22 μm filter. Finally, add dropwise 1 mL of 2× HBS buffer and incubate at room temperature for 15 min. Meanwhile, add 10 μL of 50 mM chloroquine to the Phoenix E cells in the 10 cm tissue culture dish. Add the calcium phosphate precipitate dropwise and evenly over the Phoenix E cells in the 10 cm tissue culture dish. After 6 h of incubation at 37 °C, change medium to target cell medium (RPMI 1640 medium containing 20% FCS, 1% penicillin/streptomycin, and 2 mM L-glutamine) and incubate at 37 °C for 48 h.

Day -2: Transfection efficiency is estimated via fluorescence microscopy when using retroviral particles carrying a fluorescent marker. Harvest the retroviral supernatant by using a 10 mL syringe and filter through a 0.45 μm filter. Use the retroviral supernatant for transduction of bone marrow cells on day -2 (*see* Subheading 3.4). Add target cell medium to the Phoenix E cells again and incubate at 37 °C for another 24 h.

Day -1: Harvest the retroviral supernatant and filter through a 0.45 μm filter. Use the retroviral supernatant for transduction of bone marrow cells on day -1 (*see* Subheading 3.4).

3.3 Isolation of Bone Marrow Cells

Day -3: Euthanize donor mice, collect femur and tibia of both legs, and remove termini at the epiphyses. Use a 22 G needle fitted on a 5 mL syringe filled with RPMI 1640 medium (containing 10% FCS, 1% penicillin/streptomycin, and 2 mM L-glutamine) to flush the marrow through a 40 μm cell strainer into a 15 mL conical tube. Keep isolated cells on ice. Centrifuge bone marrow cells (400 g, 5 min, 4 °C) and resuspend them in red blood cell lysis buffer to lyse bone marrow erythrocytes according to the manufacturer's protocol. Stop lysis after 5 min, centrifuge cells again (400 g, 5 min, 4 °C), and count them by using a hemocytometer. Resuspend cells in RPMI 1640 medium (containing 20% FCS, 1% penicillin/streptomycin, 2 mM L-glutamine, 10 ng/mL recombinant murine IL 3, 10 ng/mL recombinant murine IL 6, and 100 ng/mL recombinant murine SCF). Seed 3×10^6 nucleated cells in 1 ml medium per well of a 12-well cell culture plate and culture them at 37 °C overnight (*see* **Note 5**).

3.4 Transduction of Bone Marrow Cells

Day -2: Monitor growth of cultured bone marrow cells under a light microscope (*see* **Note 5**). Prior to transduction, add 10 ng/mL recombinant murine IL 3, 10 ng/mL recombinant murine IL 6, 100 ng/mL recombinant murine SCF, and

4 μg/mL polybrene to the freshly harvested and filtered retroviral supernatant. For transduction, add 2 mL of retroviral supernatant per well of cultured bone marrow cells. Incubate at 37 °C overnight.

Day -1: Monitor growth of cultured bone marrow cells under a light microscope again (*see* **Note 5**). Centrifuge bone marrow cells (400 g, 5 min, room temp.). Aspirate old supernatant and add another 2 mL of freshly harvested and filtered retroviral supernatant (containing recombinant murine IL 3, IL 6, SCF, and polybrene) per well of cultured bone marrow cells. Incubate at 37 °C overnight.

3.5 Stem Cell Transplantation

Day 0: Centrifuge bone marrow cells (400 g, 5 min, 4 °C). Aspirate supernatant and resuspend cells in 5 mL PBS. Repeat centrifugation and aspiration twice to remove FCS. Keep cells on ice. Count cells by using a hemocytometer and determine the transduction efficiency via flow cytometry (*see* **Notes 6** and 7). Use an x-ray or γ-ray radiation source for lethal whole-body irradiation (9 Gy) of 6–8-week-old isogenic recipient mice. For the irradiation procedure, keep the mice inside an irradiation box without fixation. Four hours after irradiation, fix single mice inside a mouse restrainer and intravenously (i.v.) inject transduced and nontransduced bone marrow cells (0.5×10^6 cells resuspended in 250 μL PBS per recipient mouse, 5–20% transduced cells, and 80–95% non-transduced cells) (*see* **Note 7**) into the tail vein of the recipient mice by using a 26 G needle fitted on a 1 mL syringe. Transfer of nontransduced bone marrow cells is necessary to provide some hematopoietic function in the completely myeloablated recipient mice [2, 4].

3.6 Analysis

Monitor weight of the mice and look for clinical symptoms of leukemia. Periodically sample peripheral blood from the tail vein and determine white blood cell count and the number of fluorescently labeled leukemic cells via flow cytometry to track reconstitution of the hematopoietic system and leukemic progression. Mice exhibiting severe symptoms of sickness (weight loss, rough hair coat, lethargy) should be euthanized. Peripheral blood, spleen, liver, and bone marrow can be harvested, and weight and size of the organs should be determined. Further analysis of these organs via flow cytometry is recommended [5]. Alternatively, leukemic mice can be treated with cancer therapeutics and used for studying new treatment regimens.

4 Notes

1. Phoenix E cells are recommended for retroviral transfection as they are characterized by expression of *env* and *gag-pol* genes necessary for retroviral particle production.
2. Use a retrovirus carrying a fluorescent marker for later analysis via fluorescence microscopy (estimation of transfection efficiency of Phoenix E cells) and flow cytometry (determination of transduction efficiency of murine bone marrow cells).
3. Avoid repeated freeze/thaw cycles of recombinant murine IL 3, IL 6, and SCF.
4. For optimal transfection efficiency, Phoenix E cells should reach 70–80% confluency. Therefore, periodically monitor confluency prior to transfection. If confluency is lower than 70–80%, culture the cells for another 6–12 h and periodically determine confluency again. Confluency higher than 80% will also lead to a reduction in transfection efficiency.
5. The transduction efficiency of cultured bone marrow cells depends on retroviral titer and optimal target cell growth. Determination of retroviral titer is essential when transduction efficiency is too low and should be performed according to standard molecular biology protocols [4]. Insufficient cell growth can arise due to dysfunctional cytokines (recombinant murine IL 3, IL 6, and SCF) or low seeding density. Therefore, avoid repeated freeze/thaw cycles of the cytokines, seed the isolated bone marrow cells at a sufficient density (3×10^6 nucleated cells in 1 mL medium per well of a 12-well cell culture plate), and periodically monitor their growth under a light microscope. The total cell number should substantially increase during cell culture.
6. Efficient hematopoietic reconstitution depends on successful tail vein injection of murine hematopoietic cells (especially LT-HSCs) and complete myeloablation of the recipient mice. Before i.v. injection, cultured bone marrow cells can be examined for presence of hematopoietic stem and progenitor cells (HSPCs) via flow cytometry [5].
7. In our hands, a transduction efficiency of 5–20% is optimal in terms of engraftment and time of leukemic progression. Adoptive transfer of nontransduced bone marrow cells is necessary to provide some hematopoietic function in the completely myeloablated recipient mice [2, 4].

Acknowledgments

This work was supported by the Austrian Federal Ministry of Education, Science, and Research (BMBWF).

References

1. Almosailleakh M, Schwaller J (2019) Murine models of acute myeloid leukaemia. Int J Mol Sci 20. https://doi.org/10.3390/ijms20020453
2. Hemann M (2015) Reconstitution of mice with modified hematopoietic stem cells. Cold Spring Harb Protoc 2015:679–685. https://doi.org/10.1101/pdb.prot077990
3. Swift S, Lorens J, Achacoso P et al (1999) Rapid production of retroviruses for efficient gene delivery to mammalian cells using 293 T cell–based systems. Curr Protoc Immunol 31. https://doi.org/10.1002/0471142735.im1017cs31
4. Qu J, Yang Z (2021) Protocol to produce high-titer retrovirus for transduction of mouse bone marrow cells. STAR Protoc 2. https://doi.org/10.1016/j.xpro.2021.100459
5. Höckendorf U, Yabal M, Herold T et al (2016) RIPK3 restricts myeloid leukemogenesis by promoting cell death and differentiation of leukemia initiating cells. Cancer Cell 30:75–91. https://doi.org/10.1016/j.ccell.2016.06.002

Chapter 2

NOTCH1-Induced T-Cell Acute Lymphoblastic Leukemia In Vivo Models

Anna Campagnari and Laura Belver

Abstract

T-cell acute lymphoblastic leukemia (T-ALL) is primarily a NOTCH1-driven disease, which represents approximately 15% of pediatric and 25% of adult newly diagnosed ALL cases. Gain-of-function NOTCH1 mutations are highly prevalent in T-ALL contributing to almost 60% of the cases. The protocol presented here describes a method for in vivo T-ALL transformation driven by the retroviral transduction of hematopoietic progenitors with oncogenic mutant forms NOTCH1 and subsequent transplant into recipient mice. This T-ALL transformation model allows the interaction between the leukemia cells and the bone marrow microenvironment, better recapitulating the physiological conditions that promote the development of the human disease, providing a versatile tool for both experimental therapeutics and functional genetics studies on T-ALL.

Key words T-cell acute lymphoblastic leukemia (T-ALL), NOTCH1, Leukemogenesis, Mouse models, Hematopoietic progenitors, Retroviral transduction, Bone marrow transplant

1 Introduction

T-cell acute lymphoblastic leukemia (T-ALL) is a hematological tumor characterized by infiltration in the bone marrow of transformed hematopoietic cells expressing immature T-cell markers. T-ALL represents 15% of pediatric and 25% of adult cases of ALL, and it is more prevalent in males than in females (2:1) [1]. The clinical presentation of the disease includes elevated white cell counts in peripheral blood (hyperleukocytosis), adenopathies and splenomegaly, and symptoms related to bone marrow failure. In addition, patients at diagnosis commonly present infiltration of the central nervous system and mediastinal thymic masses [1].

T-ALL transformation develops in a sequential process in which molecular pathways controlling T-cell development are disrupted by accumulating genetic alterations that ultimately alter the normal growth, proliferation, survival, and differentiation of

Maja Čemažar, Tanja Jesenko and Urša Lampreht Tratar (eds.), *Mouse Models of Cancer: Methods and Protocols*,
Methods in Molecular Biology, vol. 2773, https://doi.org/10.1007/978-1-0716-3714-2_2,
© The Author(s), under exclusive license to Springer Science+Business Media, LLC, part of Springer Nature 2024

thymocytes [1]. The close relationship between the regulatory pathways controlling T-cell differentiation and the oncogenic signals driving T-ALL transformation is best illustrated by the remarkable role of NOTCH1 in both processes, as a key T-cell fate specification and development factor, and as one of the most prominent driver genes in T-ALL [1].

NOTCH1 is a class I transmembrane glycoprotein that is constitutively activated by oncogenic gain-of-function mutations in more than 60% of T-ALL patients [1]. In physiological conditions, the interaction of NOTCH1 with its ligands triggers two consecutive cleavages, first at the extracellular Heterodimerization Domain (HD) by the metalloproteinase ADAM10, and then at the transmembrane domain by the γ-secretase complex, resulting in the cytoplasmatic release of the intracellular portion of NOTCH1 (ICN1) (Fig. 1) [2]. ICN1 is then translocated to the nucleus where it associates with RBPJ and MAML1 to form a DNA-binding complex that activates a broad transcriptional program (Fig. 1) [2]. NOTCH1 signaling is ultimately terminated by the ubiquitination of the ICN1 proline (P)/glutamic acid (E)/serine (S)/threonine (T)-enriched domain (PEST) by the ubiquitin ligase FBXW7, which promotes proteasome degradation (Fig. 1) [2].

The aberrant activation of NOTCH1 in T-ALL was first identified as a rare event in patients harboring the t(7;9)(q34;q34.3) chromosomal translocation, which results in a truncated and constitutively active oncoprotein lacking the extracellular region of NOTCH1 [3]. After that initial discovery, activating mutations at the HD and the PEST domains were described in approximately two out of three T-ALL patients [4]. While HD mutations perturb NOTCH1 signaling initiation by allowing ligand-independent activation, the PEST mutations impair signaling termination by preventing proteasomal degradation due to the loss of the degron domain [4].

The oncogenic role of NOTCH1 in T-ALL was ultimately demonstrated using in vivo mouse models in which the transplantation of isogenic hematopoietic progenitors overexpressing NOTCH1 mutant forms was enough to drive T-ALL leukemogenesis. Rapid leukemia onset was reported upon expression of ICN1 or ΔE-NOTCH1 (a truncated NOTCH1 receptor lacking the extracellular portion) in murine hematopoietic progenitors (Fig. 2) [5]. These NOTCH1 oncogenic mutants are found in only 1% of T-ALL patients and recapitulate very aggressive forms of the disease in mice. Alternatively, mice transplanted with NOTCH1 forms harboring mutations at the HD and the PEST domains, which co-occur in around 20% of T-ALL patients, developed a less aggressive disease with longer latency, which better resembles the human disease, and suggests a correlation between

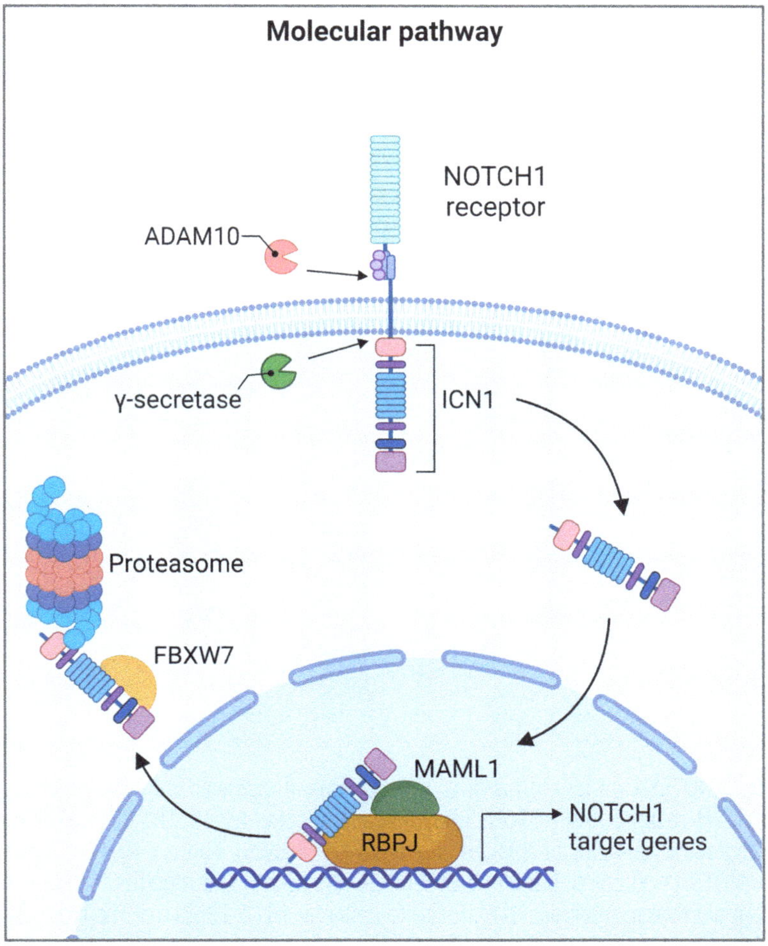

Fig. 1 The NOTCH1 signaling pathway. NOTCH1 is a single-pass type I transmembrane receptor. Signal transduction through NOTCH1 requires the extracellular engagement of the receptor with specific ligands that trigger first the cleavage of the extracellular part of NOTCH1 at the heterodimerization domain (HD) by the metalloproteinase ADAM10, and then an intracellular cleavage by the γ-secretase complex, which releases the active intracellular domains of NOTCH1 (ICN1) to the cytoplasm. ICN1 is then translocated to the nucleus where it interacts with RBPJ and MALM1 to form a DNA-binding complex that activates a broad transcriptional program regulating cell growth and metabolism. NOTCH1 signal transduction termination requires the phosphorylation of the ICN1 PEST domain and consequent ubiquitination by FBXW7, leading to proteasome degradation

degree of pathway activation and leukemic development (Fig. 2) [6].

The following protocol outlines a method to efficiently transduce murine hematopoietic progenitors with retroviral vectors encoding oncogenic NOTCH1 forms and the transplant of these

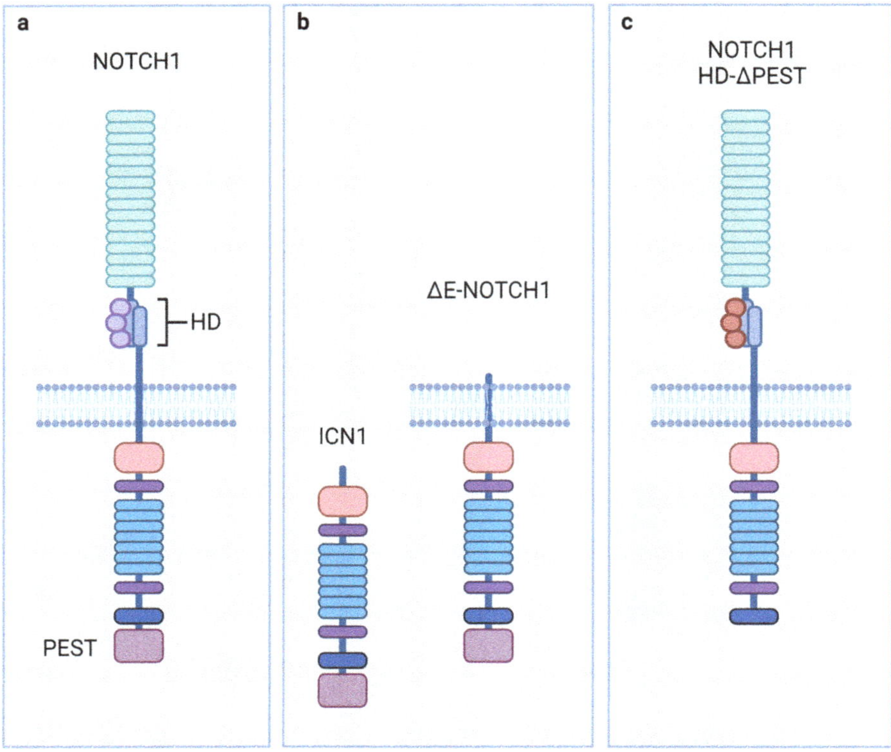

Fig. 2 NOTCH1 mutant forms driving T-ALL leukemogenesis in in vivo models. (**a**) Membrane bound wild-type NOTCH1 receptor. (**b**) NOTCH1 intracellular truncated forms. The ICN1 protein is compound of only the active cytoplasmic domains of NOTCH1 (residues 1770-2555). The ΔE-NOTCH1 protein also contains the intracellular NOTCH1 domains, but it is bound to the membrane and requires the cleavage by the γ-secretase complex to get activated (residues 1-22 fused to residues 1673-2555). (**c**) The NOTCH1-HD-ΔPEST protein contains a mutation at the HD domain (L1601P) and a frameshift mutation that truncates the PEST domain (residues 2473-2555). These mutations allow a ligand-independent activation of NOTCH1 and prevent protein degradation, respectively

cells into isogenic recipient mice, as a model to reproduce T-ALL leukemogenesis *in vivo* (Fig. 3). This approach provides a useful experimental platform to assess the efficacy of drugs for the treatment of T-ALL. Moreover, the combination of this protocol with hematopoietic precursor from genetically-modified donor animals is a valuable tool to study the contribution specific genetic alterations to leukemia initiation and/or progression.

2 Materials

2.1 Retroviral Supernatant Preparation

1. HEK-293 T cells.
2. Cell culture dishes (100 mm or 150 mm).
3. 0.25% trypsin solution.

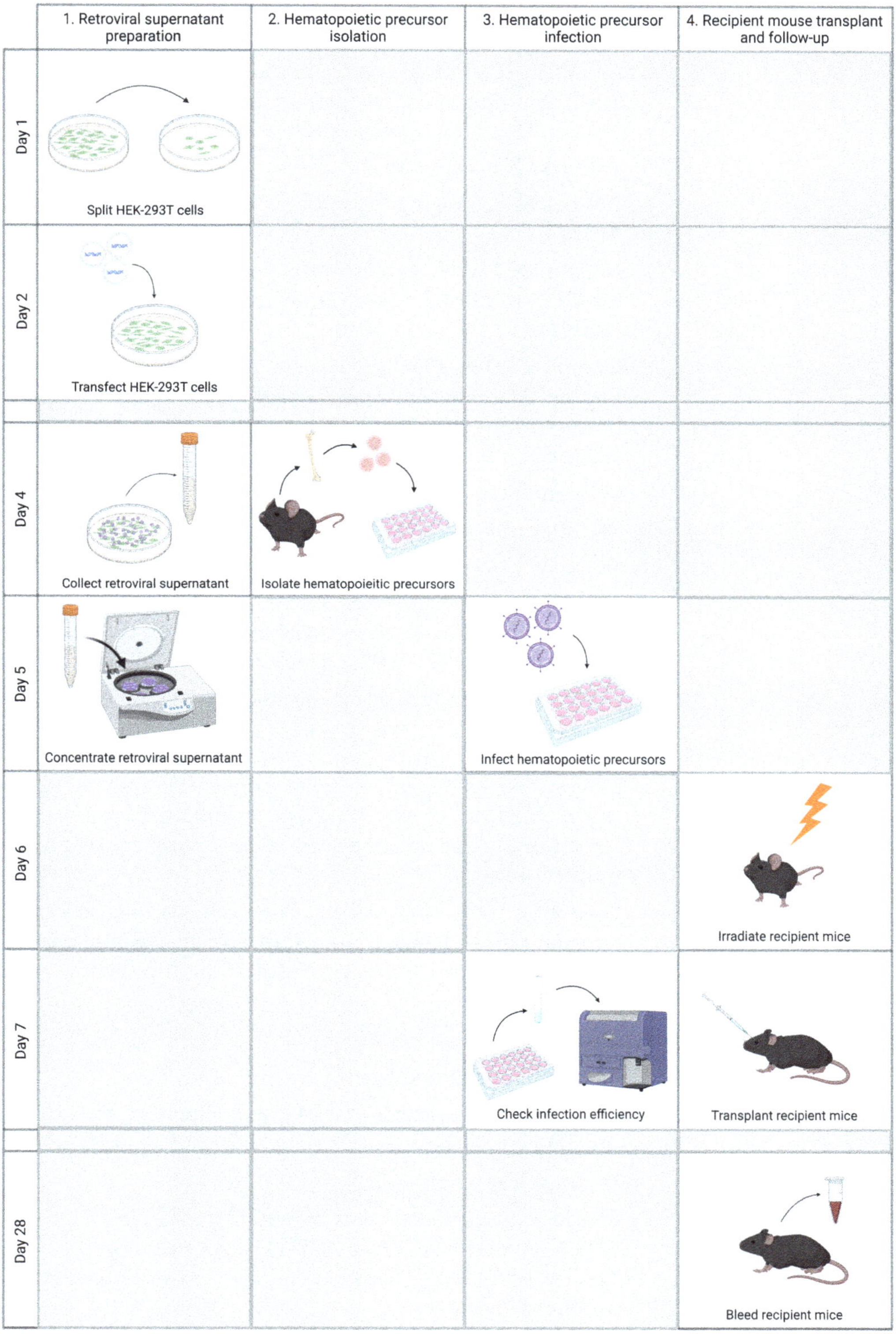

Fig. 3 Schematic overview of the experimental design. Columns represent the four work packages from the Methods section. Rows show the daily schedule for each specific task of the work packages

4. PEI MAX® -Transfection Grade Linear Polyethylenimine Hydrochloride, Molecular Weight 40 kDa (CAS number 49553-93-7—Polysciences, catalog number 24765-100). Stock solution must be prepared following manufacturer's protocol at a final concentration of 1 mg/mL in sterile water.
5. 150 mM NaCl solution.
6. Retrovirus packaging plasmid pCL-Eco (AddGene Plasmid #12371).
7. Mutant *NOTCH1*-expressing retroviral vector encoding also for GFP or other flow cytometry trackable fluorescent protein (*see* **Note 1**).
8. Complete HEK-293 T cell culture media: Dulbecco's Modified Eagle's Medium (DMEM), supplemented with 10% fetal bovine serum (FBS) and 1% penicillin–streptomycin solution (10,000 U/mL) (Pen-Strep).
9. 0.45 μm filters.
10. 20, 30, or 50 mL syringes, as required.
11. Retro-X Concentrator™ supernatant concentration reagent (Takara, catalog number 631456).
12. Retroviral supernatant resuspension media: Opti-MEM™ supplemented with 10% FBS and 1% Pen-Strep.
13. Polybrene (hexadimethrine bromide—CAS number 28728-55-4).

2.2 Hematopoietic Precursor Isolation

1. Donor mice: 6–8-week-old mice from a wild-type background (*e.g.*, C57BL/6) or harboring a genetic modification of interest (*see* **Note 2**). Use one donor mouse to transplant two to three recipient mice.
2. Dissection tools: fine scissors, bone scissors, fine forceps (for skin and muscle removal, tip width approx. 0.8 mm), and two standard forceps (for bone dislocation, tip width approx. 2.5 mm).
3. Carbon steel razor blades.
4. Porcelain mortar and pestle.
5. Bone processing media: DMEM, supplemented with 10% FBS and 1% Pen-Strep.
6. 70 μm cell strainers.
7. Red Blood Cell (RBC) lysis buffer: 150 mM NH_4Cl, 0.1 mM EDTA, 10 mM $KHCO_3$ in milli-Q water. Adjust pH to 7.4 and sterilize by filtering. This buffer can be also purchased from commercial vendors.
8. Neubauer counting chamber and 0.4% Trypan Blue Solution, or other cell counting system.

9. Murine lineage cell depletion kit (Miltenyi Biotec, catalog number 130-090-858).
10. Isolation buffer: 1× phosphate-buffered saline (PBS), 0.5% bovine serum albumin (BSA), and 2 mM EDTA.
11. LS MACS® columns (Miltenyi Biotec, catalog number 130-042-401) (*see* **Note 3**).
12. MACS® separator system compatible with LS MACS® columns (*see* **Note 3**).
13. Complete hematopoietic precursor culture media: Opti-MEM™ supplemented with 10% FBS, 1% Pen-Strep, and the following recombinant murine cytokines: 10 ng/mL Interleukin-3 (mIL3), 10 ng/mL Interleukin-6 (mIL6), 50 ng/mL Stem Cell Factor (mSCF), 25 ng/mL Interleukin-7 (mIL7), and 50 ng/mL FMS-like Tyrosine Kinase 3 Ligand (mFLT3-L) (PreproTech, catalog numbers 213-13, 216-16, 250-03, 21717, and 250-31L, respectively).

2.3 Hematopoietic Precursor Infection

1. Hematopoietic precursor culture (from Subheading 2.2).
2. Concentrated retroviral supernatants (from Subheading 2.1).
3. Anti-mouse Ly-6A/E (Sca-1) antibody for flow cytometry (such as eBioscience APC-conjugated anti-mouse Ly-6A/E (Sca-1) antibody, catalog number 17-5981) (*see* **Note 4**).
4. Flow cytometry buffer: 1× PBS supplemented with 2% FBS or BSA.
5. Flow cytometer (*see* **Note 4**).
6. Sterile 1× PBS.

2.4 Recipient Mouse Transplant and Follow-Up

1. Recipient mice: 6–8-week-old mice with the same genetic background as the donor mice (*see* **Note 2**).
2. Small animal irradiator.
3. Isoflurane anesthesia chamber.
4. 0.5% proparacaine hydrochloride ophthalmic solution.
5. Sterile 1× PBS.
6. 1 mL low dead space syringes and 26 Gauge needles.
7. 0.25 mg/mL enrofloxacin, dissolved in sterile tap water (do not use deionized water).
8. Single-use sterile lancet (5 mm).
9. Heparin or EDTA blood collection microtubes.
10. RBC lysis buffer (as in Subheading 2.2).
11. Flow cytometry buffer (as in Subheading 2.3).
12. Anti-mouse CD4 and anti-mouse CD8a antibodies for flow cytometry (such as BD Pharmingen APC-Cy7-conjugated

anti-mouse CD4 antibody, catalog number 552051, and eBioscience PE-Cy7 anti-mouse CD8a antibody, catalog number 25-0081) (*see* **Note 4**).

3 Methods

3.1 Retroviral Supernatant Preparation

1. Grow HEK-293 T cells in complete HEK-293 T cell culture media on a tissue culture dish (100 mm or 150 mm) to confluence (80–90% coverage).

Day 1

2. Add 0.25% trypsin solution to confluent HEK-293 T cell plates (5 mL to 100 mm dishes and 10 mL to 150 mm dishes) and incubate at room temperature for 30 s. Aspirate the trypsin solution, and detach HEK-293 T cells from the dish surface using complete HEK-293 T cell culture media (5 mL for 100 mm dishes and 10 mL for 150 mm dishes). Resuspend by pipetting up and down to obtain and homogeneous cell suspension and split the cells in fresh tissue culture dishes (1:5 dilution). The number and size of dishes needed will depend on the number of animals to be transplanted (*see* **Note 5**).

Day 2

3. Prepare transfection mix A by combining PEI MAX® stock solution with 150 mM NaCl solution:
   - For 150 mm dish: add 75 μL of PEI MAX® stock solution to 425 μL of 150 mM NaCl solution.
   - For 100 mm dish: add 30 μL of PEI MAX® stock solution to 220 μL of 150 mM NaCl solution.

   Incubate mix A for 5 min at room temperature.
4. Prepare mix B combining pCL-Eco and mutant *NOTCH1*-encoding plasmid with 150 mM NaCl solution:
   - For 150 mm dish: add 10 μg of pCL-Eco and 10 μg of *NOTCH1*-encoding plasmid to 500 μL of 150 mM NaCl solution.
   - For 100 mm dish: add 5 μg of pCL-Eco and 5 μg of *NOTCH1*-encoding plasmid to 250 μL of 150 mM NaCl solution.
5. Prepare transfection mix by combining mix A and mix B. Notice that, while the volume of mix A will be always constant (500 μL for a 150 mm dish and 250 for a 100 mm

dish), mix B volume will vary depending on the plasmid concentrations. It is recommended to use plasmid stock concentrations ≥1 μg/μL, which will result in mix B volumes of 500–520 μL for a 150 mm dish and 250–260 μL for a 100 mm dish. However, mix A and mix B volumes must be combined in full, independently of these small variations.

6. Vortex transfection mix (mix A + mix B) vigorously and incubate for 15 min.
7. Add the full volume of the transfection mix (approximately 1 mL for 150 mm dishes and 500 μL for 100 mm dishes) dropwise on HEK-293 T cells while rocking the dish. Incubate in standard conditions for 48 h.

Day 4

8. Collect retroviral supernatant and filter it through a 0.45 μm using a syringe. Do not extract the plunger of the syringe while attached to the filter. Use a syringe size that fits the total volume of supernatant or several syringes and filters. Reusing is not recommended. All the material that is in contact with the retroviral supernatant should be bleached before disposing.
9. Optional: It is recommended to check HEK-293 T transfection efficiency by flow cytometry or fluorescence microscopy.
10. Add Retro-X Concentrator™ reagent to the filtered retroviral supernatant following manufacturer's protocol and incubate at 4 °C overnight.

Day 5

11. Centrifuge the Retro-X Concentrator™/retroviral supernatant mix at 1500× g for 45 min at 4 °C.
12. Discard supernatant carefully and resuspend pellet in retroviral supernatant resuspension media to achieve a 3× concentrated supernatant (*e.g.*, if starting from 30 mL of non-concentrated supernatant, resuspend pellet in 10 mL of resuspension media).
13. Add polybrene to a final concentration of 8 μg/mL.

3.2 Hematopoietic Precursor Isolation

Day 4

1. Euthanize donor mice by cervical dislocation and place them onto a sterile surgical pad in a sterile environment. Sterilize mouse abdomen and limb skin areas with 70% ethanol.

2. Dissect donor mice to obtain limb bones (*i.e.*, femurs, tibiae, humeri, radii, and ulnae) and hip bones. Remove the muscles and residue tissues surrounding the bones using a razor blade.
3. Place clean bones in a mortar in bone processing media and crash them with the pestle.
4. Filter bone processing media through a 70 μm cell strainer placed on a 50 mL conical tube to obtain a single-cell suspension. Crashed bones should look white at this point. If they are still red in some areas, it is possible to perform a second round of crashing and filtering to maximize the number of cells recovered.
5. Centrifuge 5 min at 500× g and discard the supernatant carefully and add 2 mL of RBC lysis buffer per donor mouse. Incubate for 5 min.
6. Wash by adding 5 volumes of bone processing media and centrifuge 5 min at 500× g.
7. Discard supernatant, resuspend cell pellet in isolation buffer (10 mL per donor mouse), and count the number of recovered cells.
8. Isolate hematopoietic progenitors by using the murine lineage cell depletion kit following manufacturer's protocol.
9. Count isolated hematopoietic progenitors and plate in 24-well plates (2 mL per well) at a concentration of 1×10^6 cells/mL in complete hematopoietic precursor culture media. Incubate in standard conditions for 24 h.

3.3 Hematopoietic Precursor Infection

Day 5

1. Carefully remove the media from the hematopoietic precursor cultures without disturbing the cells and save it in a conical tube at 4 °C.
2. Add 1 mL of concentrated retroviral supernatant to each well.
3. Spin for 90 min at 1300× g and room temperature.
4. Incubate cells in standard conditions for at least 6 h.
5. Remove retroviral supernatant and replace it with previously saved hematopoietic precursor culture media. Culture cells in standard conditions for 48 h.

Day 7

6. Resuspend the cells in their own culture media by pipetting and pool them in a conical tube. Take a 200 μL aliquot for flow cytometry analysis.

7. Spin the cell aliquot for 5 min at 500× g and stain the pelleted cells with a fluorochrome-conjugated anti-mouse Ly-6A/E (Sca-1) antibody (*see* **Note 4**) in flow cytometry buffer for 20 min on ice and protected from light.
8. Wash cells with flow cytometry buffer and spin for 5 min at 500× g.
9. Resuspend cells in 300 μL flow cytometry buffer for analysis.
10. Determined the percentage of infected Ly-6A/E (Sca-1) in the culture (double positive for Ly-6A/E (Sca-1) and GFP or equivalent retrovirally-expressed fluorescent protein).
11. Count pooled cells from step 6 and calculate the absolute number of infected Ly-6A/E (Sca-1) cells.
12. Spin cells as in step 7 and resuspend in sterile 1× PBS to achieve a concentration of 0.5 million of infected Ly-6A/E (Sca-1) cells per mL. Use this cell suspension to transplant host animals (Subheading 3.4, **step 3**).

3.4 Recipient Mouse Transplant and Follow-Up

Day 6

1. Perform sublethal irradiation (2 Gy) on restrained recipient animals (*see* **Note 6**).

Day 7

2. Anesthetize recipient mice in an isoflurane chamber (4.5% isoflurane). The level of anesthesia induction can be verified by monitoring the loss of the foot retraction reflex in response to the stimulus.
3. Place anesthetized mice onto a sterile surgical pad in a sterile environment. Apply one drop of proparacaine solution on the eye and inject 100 μL of cell suspension (prepared in Subheading 3.3, **step 12**) via retro-orbital injection, using a 1 mL syringe with a 26 G needle (*see* **Note 7**).
4. After injection, place transplanted mice in a clean, dry, quiet environment away from other animals, and visually monitor anesthesia recovery. Motor and sensory functions recovered within minutes after termination of isoflurane administration. Once the mice can maintain upright posture and walk normally, they can be return to the animal housing room.
5. Provide transplanted animals with enrofloxacin 0.25 mg/mL in water ad libitum for 2 weeks after transplantation to prevent possible infections derived from the procedure and follow-up (*see* **Note 8**).

Day 28

6. Bleed mice by submandibular puncture with a sterile 5 mm lancet on heparin or EDTA-coated tubes (maximum of 100 μL per animal).
7. Resuspend blood samples in 1 mL of RBC lysis buffer and incubate 5 min at room temperature. Wash by adding 5 volumes of flow cytometry buffer and centrifuge 5 min at 500× g. Discard supernatant.
8. Repeat **step** 7 (RBC lysis + washing) two additional times.
9. Stain the pelleted cells with fluorochrome-conjugated anti-mouse CD4 and CD8a antibodies (*see* **Note 4**) in flow cytometry buffer for 20 min on ice and protected from light.
10. Wash cells with 500 μL flow cytometry buffer and centrifuge 5 min at 500× g.
11. Resuspend cells in 300 μL flow cytometry buffer for analysis.
12. Determine the percentage of CD4/CD8a double positive cells in circulation (*see* **Note 9**).
13. Monitor the animals periodically (*see* **Note 10**).

4 Notes

1. T-ALL induction using this protocol can be driven by the overexpression of different *NOTCH1* mutant forms. The most prominent oncogenic effects are achieved using retroviruses encoding for either the cytoplasmic intracellular portion of NOTCH1 (ICN1, residues 1770 through 2555) or the membrane-bound protein (ΔE-NOTCH1, residues 1 through 22 fused to residues 1673 through 2555) (Fig. 2) [5, 7]. These mutant forms are observed in only 1% of T-ALL patients and occur due to a rare chromosomal rearrangement (the t(7;9)(q34;q34.3) translocation) that results in high levels of expression of the truncated receptor [3, 8]. While ICN1 does not need any processing to trigger NOTCH1 signaling, ΔE-NOTCH1 needs to be cleaved from the membrane by the γ-secretase complex to release the active ICN1 domain. It is for this reason that, although both ICN1 and ΔE-NOTCH1 induce T-ALL with a 100% penetrance, the latency is significantly reduced in the case of ICN1-infected hematopoietic progenitors (approximately 6 weeks) when compared to ΔE-NOTCH1 (8–10 weeks).

   Alternatively, another mutant NOTCH1 receptor commonly used in T-ALL induction assays is the NOTCH1-HD-

ΔPEST. Gain-of-function mutations at the HD or the PEST domains account for more than 60% of T-ALL cases. Moreover, co-occurrence of these two genetic alterations is present in approximately 20% of the patients [4]. Thus, the NOTCH1-HD-ΔPEST receptor better resembles the most frequent mutations observed in human T-ALL by harboring a point mutation at the HD domain (L1601P) that allows ligand-independent NOTCH1 activation, and a frameshift mutation that truncates the PEST domain (residues 2473 through 2555), which is involved in the proteolytic degradation of ICN1. The NOTCH1-HD-ΔPEST induces T-ALL with a penetrance that ranges from 60% to 80% with a latency of 3–-6 months [6]. However, it should be noted that NOTCH1 signaling is highly dose-dependent and the penetrance/latency of these assays may be affected by the levels of expression achieved in each specific experimental setting.

Another important matter to consider is that, although using ICN1 or ΔE-NOTCH1 alleles as drivers for T-ALL induction is significantly more time- and cost-efficient, the strong phenotype obtained with these mutant forms might mask the possible effects of drugs or the contribution of other mutations of interest. In those cases, in which no significant differences in the onset of the disease or the survival of the animals are observed using ICN1 and/or ΔE-NOTCH1, we recommend to use the NOTCH1-HD-ΔPEST allele, which provides a milder T-ALL phenotype that might unveil effects otherwise overlooked when using strong NOTCH1 mutant forms.

2. Donor and recipient mice must be isogenic (same genetic background) to avoid graft-versus-host and host-versus-graft responses. If this is not possible because the donor mice come from a mixed or an unknown background, an immunodeficient mouse strain, such as NOD.Cg-Prkdc^{scid} Il2rg^{tm1Wjl}/SzJ (NSG) mice (Jackson Laboratory, strain number 005557), must be used as recipient.
3. Miltenyi Biotec offers both manual and automatic magnetic depletion systems that can be used indistinctly for this purpose. In the case of manual separators, magnets that are compatible with LS MACS® columns must be chosen, such as QuadroMACS™ (catalog number 130-090-976) or MidiMACS™ (catalog number 130-042-302), to be used in combination with a MACS® MultiStand (catalog number 130-042-303). All the necessary components for manual depletion (including QuadroMACS™, MACS® MultiStand, LS MACS® Columns, and murine lineage cell depletion kit) can be also purchased together as a QuadroMACS™ Starting Kit (LS) (catalog number 130-091-051).

Alternatively, automatic magnetic depletion systems, such as autoMACS® Pro Separator (catalog number 130-092-545), can also be used in this protocol. If opting for automatic depletion, LS MACS® Columns will not be required, but other consumables will be necessary for operating the equipment as described by the manufacturer.

Finally, although Miltenyi Biotec is the gold standard for magnetic depletion, other companies offer similar systems that might be used in this protocol, although the use of these alternatives might affect the recovery and purity of the isolated hematopoietic progenitors.

4. The fluorochrome-conjugated antibodies suggested in this protocol are just illustrative examples. The antibody selection must be done taking into account both the fluorescent protein expressed by vector that will be used for the retroviral infections, and the laser and filter configuration of the cytometer. Thus, the excitation/emission spectrum of the fluorochromes conjugated to the antibodies must be compatible with the one of the fluorescent protein expressed by the cells, and all of them must be detectable by the available cytometer.

5. The number and size of the plates needed for transfection will depend on the number of bone marrow donor animals required for the experiment. After hematopoietic precursor isolation, around 2 million cells will be recovered from each 6- to 8-week-old donor mouse (using both leg and arm bones), which should be enough to transplant two to three recipient mice. Before infection, purified hematopoietic progenitors are cultured in 24-well plates (2 mL per well) at a concentration of 1×10^6 cells/mL (approximately one well per donor mouse). Each of these wells will require 1 mL of 3× concentrated retroviral supernatant for infection. Thus, 3 mL of non-concentrated retroviral supernatant must be prepared per well of hematopoietic progenitors. Taking this into account, 100 mm and 150 mm plates can produce approximately 10 mL and 25 mL of nonconcentrated retroviral supernatant, respectively. These volumes should be enough to infect approximately three wells in the case of 100 mm plates and eight in the case of 150 mm plates after 3x concentration.

   Practical example:

   - Number of recipient animals: 20.
   - Number of donor animals needed to transplant 20 recipient mice: 7–10.
   - Expected number of hematopoietic progenitors recovered from the donor mice after isolation: 14–20 million cells.
   - Number of wells (24-well plate) required for hematopoietic precursor culture before infection: 7–10 wells.

- Amount of 3× concentrated retroviral supernatant required for the infection: 7–10 mL.
- Amount of nonconcentrated retroviral supernatant required for the infection: 21–30 mL.
- Recommended number and size of plates for retroviral supernatant production: three 100 mm plates.

6. The effects derived from the irradiation may vary between different irradiators and mouse strains. For this reason, it is recommended to test the irradiation settings before performing the actual experiment. Irradiation can also be performed on the very same day of the transplant (day 7) but at least 4 h before the injection of the progenitors.
7. Resuspend the cell suspension by inversion before loading it into the syringe for injection to prevent cell sedimentation and aggregation at the bottom of the tube.
8. In the days following transplantation, the animals should be examined for signs of inflammation, conjunctivitis, blepharospasm, or other sequelae resulting from the eye trauma. If any of these conditions is detected, a veterinary evaluation should be sought to determine whether intervention or euthanasia of the affected animal is necessary.
9. Using this NOTCH1-driven T-ALL induction protocol, a transient wave of CD4/CD8a double positive cells should be observed exactly 21 days after transplant. This wave represents a preleukemic state characterized by extrathymic immature T-cell development, which precedes oncogenic transformation to T-ALL.
10. Transplanted mice must be monitored regularly considering the expected tumor latency based on the NOTCH1 mutant form that has been used to induce the disease (ICN1, ΔE-NOTCH1, or NOTCH1-HD-ΔPEST, *see* **Note 1**). The follow-up will consist of a periodical bleeding to determine by flow cytometry the percentage of fluorescent cells present in the blood (GFP or equivalent retrovirally-expressed fluorescent protein). The analysis can be performed in combination with CD4 and CD8a fluorochrome-conjugated antibodies (as described in Subheading 3.4) to establish the immunophenotype of the fluorescent cells. Alternatively, if a luciferase-expressing vector is used for the infection of the hematopoietic progenitors, leukemia progression can be monitored using an in vivo bioimaging system, such as IVIS Spectrum.

    In experimental therapeutics assays, it is recommended to start treating the animals when the tumor load in peripheral blood reaches 10–20%. Either in this case or in standard survival experiments (without treatment), the experimental endpoint must be determined by the presence of symptoms of clinically overt disease (do not feed, lack of activity, abnormal grooming behavior, hunch back posture) or excessive weight loss (>15%).

Acknowledgments

We thank the CERCA Program (Generalitat de Catalunya), the Josep Carreras Leukemia Research Institute and the Catalan Institute of Oncology for their institutional support, and the members of the Leukemia and Immuno-Oncology Group. LB is supported by the FERO Foundation (BFero2020.03), the Spanish Ministry of Science and Innovation (MCI) (PID2020-117645RB-I00/AEI/10.13039/501100011033 and RYC2020-029400-I/AEI/10.13039/501100011033), the Merck-Salud Foundation, the FEDER Foundation, and the Josep Carreras Foundation. All figures in this manuscript have been created with BioRender.

References

1. Belver L, Ferrando A (2016) The genetics and mechanisms of T cell acute lymphoblastic leukaemia. Nat Rev Cancer 16(8):494–507
2. Dumortier A, Wilson A, MacDonald HR et al (2005) Paradigms of notch signaling in mammals. Int J Hematol 82(4):277–284
3. Ellisen LW, Bird J, West DC et al (1991) *TAN-1*, the human homolog of the Drosophila *Notch* gene, is broken by chromosomal translocations in T lymphoblastic neoplasms. Cell 66(4):649–661
4. Weng AP, Ferrando AA, Lee W et al (2004) Activating mutations of NOTCH1 in human T cell acute lymphoblastic leukemia. Science 306(5694):269–271
5. Pear WS, Aster JC, Scott ML et al (1996) Exclusive development of T cell neoplasms in mice transplanted with bone marrow expressing activated Notch alleles. J Exp Med 183(5):2283–2291
6. Wendorff AA, Ferrando AA (2020) Modeling NOTCH1 driven T-cell acute lymphoblastic leukemia in mice. Bio Protoc 10(10):e3620
7. Aster JC, Robertson ES, Hasserjian RP et al (1997) Oncogenic forms of NOTCH1 lacking either the primary binding site for RBP-Jk; or nuclear localization sequences retain the ability to associate with RBP-Jk; and activate transcription *. J Biol Chem 272(17):11336–11343
8. Palomero T, Barnes KC, Real PJ et al (2006) CUTLL1, a novel human T-cell lymphoma cell line with t(7;9) rearrangement, aberrant NOTCH1 activation and high sensitivity to γ-secretase inhibitors. Leukemia 20(7):1279–1287

Chapter 3

Urinary Bladder Cancer Induced by N-Butyl-N-(4-Hydroxybutyl)-Nitrosamine

Daša Zupančič and Rok Romih

Abstract

Urinary bladder cancer is the tenth most common cancer worldwide with high morbidity and mortality. The majority of bladder cancers are urothelial carcinomas. More than half are papillomas or the papillary urothelial carcinomas (stages Ta and T1), which have a relatively good prognosis. Squamous cell carcinomas have a variable survival rate, while carcinomas in situ (Tis) can progress to muscle-invasive urothelial carcinomas (T2) with a poor prognosis. The most challenging feature of bladder cancer is its high recurrence rate, ranging from 50% to 90% of cases. The N-butyl-N-(4-hydroxybutyl)-nitrosamine (BBN) model is an invaluable experimental tool for bladder cancer research, as BBN-induced bladder cancer in rodents resembles human bladder cancer in its morphological, biological, and molecular features. We present here a detailed protocol for the treatment of mice and the main expected results.

Key words Urinary bladder, Urothelium, N-butyl-N-(4-hydroxybutyl)-nitrosamine (BBN), Urinary bladder cancer, Atypia, Hyperplasia, Dysplasia, Papillary urothelial carcinoma, Invasive urothelial carcinomas

1 Introduction

Urinary bladder cancer is the most common tumor of the urinary tract. It is a heterogeneous disease with a spectrum of pathologies and clinical outcomes and is closely associated with chemical exposures, such as occupational exposure to carcinogenic aromatic amines and cigarette smoking (accounting for up to 50% of all bladder cancer diagnoses) [1]. Bladder cancer is most common in men in southern and western Europe and North America, where it is the fourth most common cancer [2]. In women, the incidence of bladder cancer is currently much lower than in men. However, it has been increasing since the mid-1990s, while it has been decreasing in men [3]. In addition, the incidence and prevalence of bladder cancer are increasing and are associated with high morbidity. The number of bladder cancer cases and deaths is expected to increase in

Maja Čemažar, Tanja Jesenko and Urša Lampreht Tratar (eds.), *Mouse Models of Cancer: Methods and Protocols*,
Methods in Molecular Biology, vol. 2773, https://doi.org/10.1007/978-1-0716-3714-2_3,
© The Author(s), under exclusive license to Springer Science+Business Media, LLC, part of Springer Nature 2024

the future due to estimated population growth and ageing, as most bladder cancer cases are diagnosed at the age of >65 years.

The majority of bladder cancers are urothelial carcinomas (90–95%), and the remainder are squamous cell carcinomas (2–5%), adenocarcinomas (0.5–2%), small cell carcinomas (<1%), and other less common malignancies. Based on the depth of invasion into the bladder wall, urothelial carcinomas can be divided into those that are confined to the urothelium (called noninvasive) and invasive. Noninvasive urothelial carcinomas are confined to the urothelium and divided into high-grade and low-grade papillary tumors (Ta) and urothelial carcinoma in situ (Tis). Tis is defined as a high-grade, flat, noninvasive lesion. Invasive urothelial carcinoma can be further subdivided into tumors that invade the lamina propria (T1) and muscularis propria (T2) or spread beyond the bladder wall into the perivesical fat tissue (T3) and sometimes into adjacent organs and/or lymph nodes (T4) [4]. For therapeutic purposes, Tis, Ta, and T1 tumors are grouped under the term nonmuscle invasive bladder cancer (NMIBC) and T2–T4 tumors under the term muscle invasive bladder cancer (MIBC). NMIBC is present in approximately 75% of patients with an initial diagnosis of bladder cancer [5]. NMIBC is usually removed by transurethral resection of the urinary bladder (TURB). Sometimes, TURB is followed by intravesical instillation of chemotherapeutic agents (mitomycin C) or Bacillus Calmette Guerin (BCG) [6]. NMIBC is characterized by an extremely high recurrence rate (50–70%), requiring systematic follow-up of patients decades after initial treatment [7]. NMIBC has a low propensity for progression (10–15%) and a 5-year survival rate of 90% [8]. The current standard treatment for MIBC is radical cystectomy, but a high rate of metastasis and a 5-year survival rate of <50% are observed [8, 9]. Due to the high recurrence rate in NMIBC and the poor survival rate in MIBC, research with reliable animal models is of utmost importance.

The most common chemical carcinogen used to cause bladder cancer is N-butyl-N-(4-hydroxybutyl)-nitrosamine (BBN) [10]. BBN is frequently found in the paint industry and is a metabolic product of various N-nitroso compounds that are also present in cigarette smoke [11]. Extensive histological [12], morphological [13], cell biological, molecular and genetic analyses [14, 15] as well as comparisons with human urothelial carcinomas [16] have been performed for the BBN-induced bladder cancer model. The major advantages of BBN are the absence of systemic toxicity and the induction of exclusively urothelial neoplasms [17], which correspond to human urothelial neoplasms in terms of onset and timing [13, 14].

The pathological and genetic similarities between the BBN-induced bladder cancer model and human disease make this model one of the most comparable systems for studying different stages of human urothelial carcinomas. As such, it supports studies on urothelial carcinoma cell biology and tumor development. The BBN-induced bladder cancer model is also very useful for evaluating new methods of treating urothelial carcinomas and for targeting drugs to cancer cells. This model is used to determine the efficacy of anticancer drugs administered to the organism intravesically (via a catheter into the urinary bladder) or by other means, e.g., orally or intraperitoneally.

BBN is administered in the form of a 0.05% solution in drinking water. Ingested BBN is metabolized in the liver, where the alcohol/aldehyde dehydrogenase enzyme system oxidizes the BBN alcohol group to the carboxyl group to form N-butyl-N-(3-carboxypropyl)-nitrosamine (BCPN). BCPN is excreted to the urine, which is stored in the bladder where it comes into contact with the urothelium. BCPN is a stable molecule that binds to urothelial cells and is directly responsible for initiating the process of cancer transformation [18]. As far as the mechanism of action is concerned, BBN belongs to the genotoxic or DNA-reactive carcinogens [19]. BBN causes damage to DNA molecules in urothelial cells and thus induces urothelial carcinogenesis [19]. The intensity of carcinogenesis and the stage at which an individual experimental animal develops bladder cancer (hyperplasia, dysplasia, Tis, low-grade noninvasive papillary urothelial carcinoma, invasive carcinoma) depends on the concentration of BBN used (besides 0.05% solution, 0.005% or 0.5% solution can also be used [15]), the duration of drinking BBN-containing water (2–24 weeks), the time interval between discontinuation of BBN water and euthanasia, collection of urothelial tissue, and the animal species and strain [20–22]. In mice, bladder changes start as an inflammatory process in the lamina propria beneath the urothelium, followed by dysplasia with urothelial metaplasia at various stages or without it, then followed by Tis and invasive carcinoma [23]. Metastases are not typical for the mouse model, as the animals are euthanized before metastases can occur due to possible obstructive uropathy.

2 Materials

1. BBN 90% stock solution (*see* **Note 1**).
2. Light-protected water bottles or aluminum foil wrapped bottles.
3. Sterile physiological solution (0.9% saline).
4. Fixatives (e.g., 4% paraformaldehyde, 10% formalin).
5. Male mice, strains A/J or C57BL/6 (*see* **Note 2**).
6. Suitable support for the mouse carcass, e.g., cork, covered with sterile foil or sterilized glass mat.

7. Sterile petri dish.
8. Sterile tweezers and scalpel.
9. Sterile glass bottles and sterile Eppendorf tubes.

3 Methods

3.1 BBN Solution

1. To obtain a 0.05% solution of BBN, add 277.7 μL of 90% BBN (stock solution) to 500 mL of tap water and mix thoroughly (*see* **Notes 3** and **4**).
2. Add 0.05% BBN to the drinking water available ad libitum to the experimental groups. Use light-protected water bottles.
3. Change 0.05% BBN in the drinking water every other day (*see* **Note 5** and **6**).

3.2 Experimental Animals

1. Randomly divide the mice into experimental groups (animals treated with 0.05% BBN for 2, 10, 15, and 17 weeks) and a control group (control animals).
2. Keep the mice in plastic cages at 23 ± 2 °C and 50–60% relative humidity in a 12-h light–dark cycle. Give all groups a standard diet available ad libitum.

3.2.1 Animals Treated with 0.05% BBN

1. Monitor health status of the mice every other day: weigh the mice, measure food and water intake (from water intake, we can also calculate the consumed amount of BBN), and observe physical appearance (e.g., fur), behavior (e.g., mobility) and reactions to external stimuli (e.g., responsiveness).
2. As there are differences both between individual animals and between different strains of mice, it is recommended to confirm the presence of tumors in mice by ultrasound during treatment.
3. Euthanize mice by CO_2 inhalation after 2, 10, 15, or 17 weeks of treatment, depending on the desired urothelial lesion to be studied (Table 1, Fig. 1).
4. Fix the mouse on a suitable support such as a cork covered with sterile foil or sterilized glass mat. Open the abdomen by making an incision in the midline. Remove the fatty tissue and viscera so that the urinary bladder is exposed and clearly visible. Lift the bladder by holding the median umbilical ligament or urachus at bladder apex with the sterile forceps and cut at the proximal part of the urethra. Cut the ligament or urachus and remove the bladder from the abdomen (*see* **Note 7**). Put the bladder on sterile petri dish, filled with sterile physiological solution.
5. Under a stereoscopic microscope, first open the bladder with sterile tweezers, then separate tumors, tumor margins, and

Table 1
Urothelial lesions in mouse carcinogenesis induced by BBN in male mice strain A/J

Weeks of BBN	Urothelial lesion
2	Urothelial atypia (100%) Desquamated urothelium (40%)
10	Hyperplasia with mild dysplasia (80%) Hyperplasia with moderate dysplasia (20%)
15	Hyperplasia with mild dysplasia (50%) Mild dysplasia without hyperplasia (50%)
17	Hyperplasia with moderate dysplasia (40%) Papillary urothelial carcinoma, low grade, invasion into lamina propria (40%) Urothelial carcinoma, low grade, invasion into lamina propria (20%)

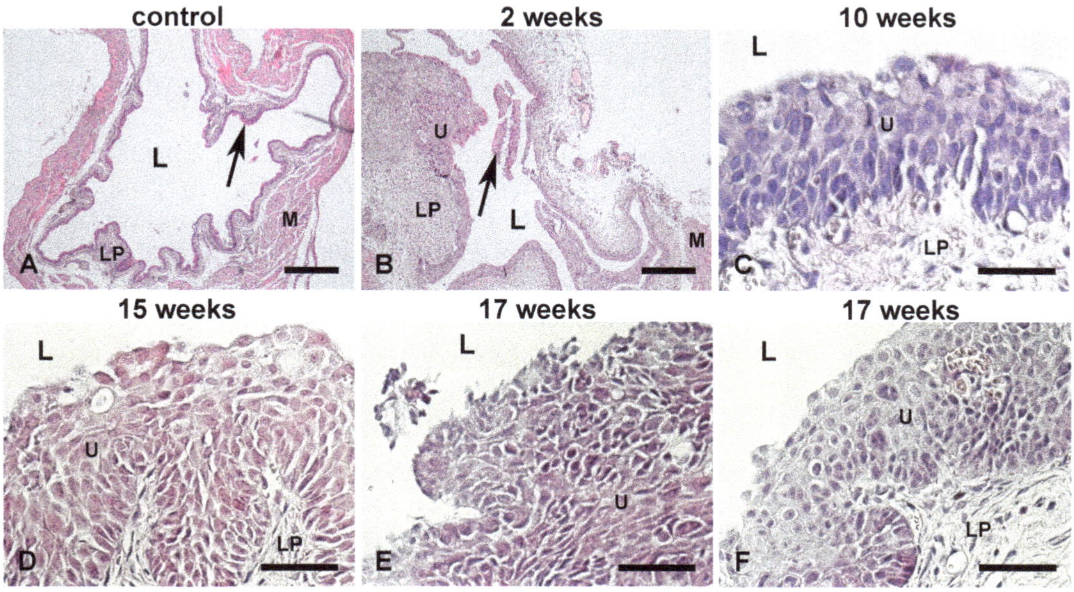

Fig. 1 Paraffin sections stained with hematoxylin and eosin of the normal urinary bladder wall of control mice (**a**) and of urothelial lesions after BBN treatment for 2 weeks (**b**), 10 weeks (**c**), 15 weeks (**d**), and 17 weeks (**e**, **f**). (**a**) The urinary bladder wall of the control mouse consists of three-layer urothelium (arrow), lamina propria (LP), and muscularis propria (M). (**b**) Urinary bladder wall (urothelium—U, lamina propria—LP, muscularis propria—M) after 2 weeks of BBN treatment showing large areas of desquamated urothelium (arrow). (**c**) Hyperplastic urothelium with mild dysplasia (U) after 10 weeks of BBN treatment. (**d**) Hyperplastic urothelium with moderate dysplasia (U) after 15 weeks of BBN treatment. (**e**, **f**) Urothelial carcinoma, low grade after 17 weeks of BBN treatment. Scale bars: A–B, 200 μm; C–F, 50 μm

normal urothelium with a scalpel. Cut each part into smaller pieces and place them in a suitable solution in sterile glass bottles or sterile Eppendorf tubes. Use sterile physiological solution for biochemical analyses (e.g., Western blot, qPCR, RNAseq) and appropriate fixative (*see* **Note 8**) for microscopy (e.g., light, fluorescence, confocal, transmission, and scanning electron microscopy).

3.2.2 Control Animals

1. The control group of mice should drink tap water without BBN for the same period as the experimental groups.
2. Weigh the mice every other day so that their health status can be monitored.
3. Repeat **steps 3–5** as described in Subheading 3.2.1.

4 Notes

1. If BBN is not used immediately store it at 4 °C in the dark. Since BBN is carcinogenic and toxic, follow the manufacturer's instructions for disposal.
2. Usually strain A/J or C57BL/6 is used, as both are well-established inbred strains. Colonies of both strains are genetically identical (when purchased from an established supplier, e.g., The Jackson Laboratories or Charles River) and have a high degree of uniformity in their inherited characteristics, or phenotypes, which include appearance, behavior, and response to experimental treatments. They have low susceptibility to spontaneous tumors and high susceptibility to tumors induced by carcinogens and are immunocompetent. Other strains of mice and also female mice can be used.
3. BBN is carcinogenic and toxic and should therefore be stored in a special place for toxic chemicals. Pipette and mix BBN in a fume hood wearing protective gloves.
4. BBN (90%) is quite viscous and difficult to pipette. We therefore recommend cutting off the tip before pipetting. Pipetting must be done slowly, and the pipette must be washed out thoroughly.
5. Always prepare 0.05% solution of BBN fresh and keep it in the dark all the time.
6. Unused BBN solution should be disposed of as hazardous waste according to the manufacturer's recommendations.
7. Dispose of the carcasses according to the legal requirements.
8. Appropriate fixatives for light microscopy are 4% paraformaldehyde or 10% formalin, for fluorescence and confocal microscopy 4% or 2% paraformaldehyde, for transmission and scanning electron microscopy the mixture of 4% paraformaldehyde and 2% glutaraldehyde.

Acknowledgments

The authors gratefully acknowledge financial support from the P3-0108, J7-2594, J3 2521, MRIC UL IP-0510 Infrastructure Programme of the Slovenian Research and Innovation Agency ARIS. We thank Sabina Železnik, Nada Pavlica Dubarić, Sanja Čabraja, and Linda Štrus for their technical support.

References

1. Magers MJ, Lopez-Beltran A, Montironi R et al (2019) Staging of bladder cancer. Histopathology 74:112–134. https://doi.org/10.1111/his.13734
2. Siegel S, Noblett K, Mangel J et al (2018) Five-year followup results of a prospective, multicenter study of patients with overactive bladder treated with sacral neuromodulation. J Urol 199:229–236. https://doi.org/10.1016/j.juro.2017.07.010
3. Antoni S, Ferlay J, Soerjomataram I et al (2017) Bladder cancer incidence and mortality: a global overview and recent trends. Eur Urol 71:96–108. https://doi.org/10.1016/j.eururo.2016.06.010
4. Amin MB, Greene FL, Edge SB et al (2017) The eighth edition AJCC cancer staging manual: continuing to build a bridge from a population-based to a more "personalized" approach to cancer staging. CA Cancer J Clin 67:93–99. https://doi.org/10.3322/caac.21388
5. Kamat AM, Hahn NM, Efstathiou JA et al (2016) Bladder cancer. Lancet 388:2796–2810. https://doi.org/10.1016/S0140-6736(16)30512-8
6. Babjuk M, Burger M, Compérat EM et al (2019) European Association of Urology guidelines on non-muscle-invasive bladder cancer (TaT1 and carcinoma in situ) – 2019 update. Eur Urol 76:639–657. https://doi.org/10.1016/j.eururo.2019.08.016
7. Ritch CR, Velasquez MC, Kwon D et al (2020) Use and validation of the AUA/SUO risk grouping for nonmuscle invasive bladder cancer in a contemporary cohort. J Urol 203:505–510. https://doi.org/10.1097/Ju.0000000000000593
8. Tan TZ, Rouanne M, Tan KT et al (2019) Molecular subtypes of urothelial bladder cancer: results from a meta-cohort analysis of 2411 tumors. Eur Urol 75:423–432. https://doi.org/10.1016/j.eururo.2018.08.027
9. Witjes JA, Bruins HM, Cathomas R et al (2021) European Association of Urology guidelines on muscle-invasive and metastatic bladder cancer: summary of the 2020 guidelines. Eur Urol 79:82–104. https://doi.org/10.1016/j.eururo.2020.03.055
10. Matsuo T, Miyata Y, Asai A et al (2017) Green tea polyphenol induces changes in cancer-related factors in an animal model of bladder cancer. PLoS One 12:e0171091. https://doi.org/10.1371/journal.pone.0171091
11. Slocum SL, Kensler TW (2011) Nrf2: control of sensitivity to carcinogens. Arch Toxicol 85:273–284. https://doi.org/10.1007/s00204-011-0675-4
12. Fukushima S, Hirose M, Tsuda H et al (1976) Histological classification of urinary bladder cancers in rats induced by N-butyl-n-(4-hydroxybutyl)nitrosamine. Gan 67:81–90
13. Gofrit ON, Birman T, Dinaburg A et al (2006) Chemically induced bladder cancer-a sonographic and morphologic description. Urology 68:231–235. https://doi.org/10.1016/j.urology.2006.03.022
14. Ariel I, Ayesh S, Gofrit O et al (2004) Gene expression in the bladder carcinoma rat model. Mol Carcinog 41:69–76. https://doi.org/10.1002/mc.20046
15. Tsuda H, Miyata Y, Hagiwara A et al (1977) Damage and repair of DNA in urinary bladder epithelium of rats treated with N-butyl-N-(4-hydroxybutyl) nitrosamine. Gan 68:781–783
16. Fantini D, Glaser AP, Rimar KJ et al (2018) A carcinogen-induced mouse model recapitulates the molecular alterations of human muscle invasive bladder cancer. Oncogene 37:1911–1925. https://doi.org/10.1038/s41388-017-0099-6
17. Bertram JS, Craig AW (1972) Specific induction of bladder cancer in mice by butyl-(4-hydroxybutyl)-nitrosamine and the effects of hormonal modifications on the sex difference in response. Eur J Cancer 8:587–594
18. Airoldi L, Magagnotti C, Bonfanti M et al (1990) Alpha-oxidative metabolism of the bladder carcinogens N-nitrosobutyl

(4-hydroxybutyl)amine and N-nitrosobutyl (3-carboxypropyl)amine within the rat isolated bladder. Carcinogenesis 11:1437–1440

19. Cohen SM (1998) Urinary bladder carcinogenesis. Toxicol Pathol 26:121–127. https://doi.org/10.1177/019262339802600114
20. Zupancic D, Korac-Prlic J, Kreft ME et al (2020) Vitamin a rich diet diminishes early urothelial carcinogenesis by altering retinoic acid signaling. Cancers (Basel) 12:1712. https://doi.org/10.3390/cancers12071712
21. Zupancic D, Kreft ME, Romih R (2014) Selective binding of lectins to normal and neoplastic urothelium in rat and mouse bladder carcinogenesis models. Protoplasma 251:49–59. https://doi.org/10.1007/s00709-013-0524-9
22. Zupančič D, Ovčak Z, Vidmar G (2011) Altered expression of UPIa, UPIb, UPII, and UPIIIa during urothelial carcinogenesis induced by N-butyl-N-(4-hydroxybutyl) nitrosamine in rats. Virchows Arch 458:603–613
23. Ohtani M, Kakizoe T, Nishio Y et al (1986) Sequential changes of mouse bladder epithelium during induction of invasive carcinomas by N-butyl-N-(4-hydroxybutyl)nitrosamine. Cancer Res 46:2001–2004

Chapter 4

Establishment of Mouse Orthotopic Urinary Bladder Tumor Model and Its Analysis by Light and Electron Microscopy

Andreja Erman, Urška Kamenšek, Dominika Peskar, and Peter Veranič

Abstract

Mouse tumor models are an important tool in cancer research, and the orthotopic cancer cell transplantation model is the most widely used among them. Methods for establishing tumor models may differ in many ways, including the selection of cancer cell lines and the type of urinary bladder pretreatment. Here, we describe our mouse orthotopic bladder tumor model using a labeled MB49 urothelial cancer cell line and chemical pretreatment with the cationic polypeptide poly-L-lysine to traumatize the bladder epithelium. Double labeling of MB49 cancer cells by their transduction with GFP and internalization of metal nanoparticles allows the study of their implantation process from the first hours to several days after intravesical injection, as well as the analysis of developed tumors after 3 weeks. Thus, our model provides a comprehensive analysis of the early and late stages of tumor development in the bladder at the light and electron microscopic level.

Key words Mouse model, Orthotopic bladder tumor model, Urinary bladder, MB49 cancer cells, Light microscopy, Electron microscopy

1 Introduction

Mouse tumor models for basic and preclinical research in bladder cancer are one of the most important oncology-related research tools. They mimic the complexity of human cancer and thus serve as a link between animal studies and clinics. There are several categories of mouse tumor models, but cancer cell line-induced models are by far the most commonly used mouse models in basic research and translational oncology [1]. In these models, tumorigenesis is characterized by the instillation of in vitro cultured cancer cell lines into mice. The models can be xenogeneic when human cancer cells are transplanted into immunocompromised mice or syngeneic when mouse cancer cells are introduced into

Maja Čemažar, Tanja Jesenko and Urša Lampreht Tratar (eds.), *Mouse Models of Cancer: Methods and Protocols*, Methods in Molecular Biology, vol. 2773, https://doi.org/10.1007/978-1-0716-3714-2_4,
© The Author(s), under exclusive license to Springer Science+Business Media, LLC, part of Springer Nature 2024

immunocompetent mice. In addition, the above two types of models can be divided into subtypes depending on the site of cancer cell transplantation. In heterotopic models, the cancer cells are implanted at a site other than the site of origin, whereas in orthotopic models, the cancer cells are implanted into the organ of origin, and thus the tumor develops orthotopically in the desired organ [1, 2]. We established an orthotopic tumor model in mice using the MB49 cancer cell line. MB49, a mouse urothelial carcinoma cell line, is one of the most commonly used murine bladder carcinoma cell lines. MB49 cancer cells are nonmuscle invasive and nonmetastatic urothelial carcinoma cells derived from carcinogen-induced mouse bladder tumors [3–7]. We have shown in our studies that MB49 cancer cells attach to the less differentiated cells of traumatized urothelium or exposed basal lamina and form tumors or hyperplastic bladder epithelium when applied to the bladder [8, 9]. It is known that traumatization of the bladder mucosa is one of the main prerequisites for the successful attachment of cancer cells and the resulting high rate of tumorigenesis [10–13]. Various techniques have been used to mechanically or chemically traumatize the bladder epithelium, called urothelium [10, 14–20]. We induced chemical injury by instilling the cationic polypeptide poly-L-lysine, which hypothetically alters the surface charges of the glycosaminoglycan layer of the urothelium and enhances the electrostatic interactions between cancer cells and normal urothelial cells [12, 13]. However, we have shown that poly-L-lysine induces intense desquamation of normal urothelial cells, resulting in partially or completely denuded areas in the urothelium where injected MB49 cancer cells can attach and implant [8, 9, 21]. Detecting MB49 cancer cells and distinguishing between cancerous urothelial cells and normal urothelial cells in vivo at the early stages of tumorigenesis were major challenges for us in developing our model. The solution was to double label MB49 cancer cells in two different ways so that they could be detected in mouse urinary bladders by light and electron microscopy. First, we prepared stable GFP-transduced MB49 cancer cells, which we observed in the urinary bladder of mice by fluorescence microscopy. We then labeled MB49-GFP cancer cells in vitro with metal nanoparticles so that they could also be identified and detected by transmission electron microscopy [9]. Here, we describe our mouse orthotopic bladder tumor model (Fig. 1), which allows us to analyze the implantation of cancer cells from very early stages of tumorigenesis (in the first hours and days after transurethral instillation of cancer cells) to fully developed bladder tumors at the optical and electron microscopic level.

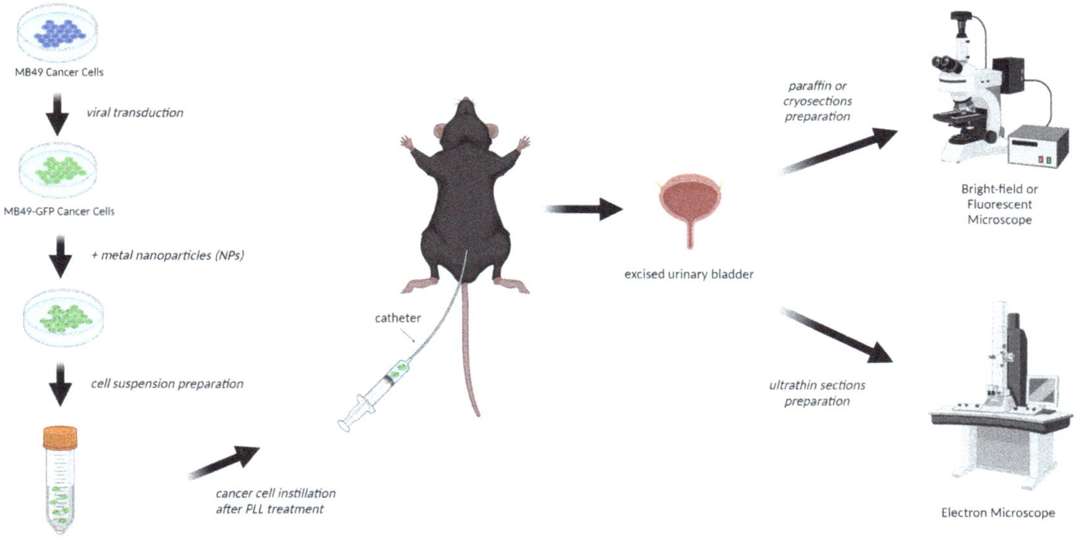

Fig. 1 Schematic protocol of the establishment and analysis of an orthotopic bladder tumor model. (Created by Biorender)

2 Materials

2.1 Materials for Cell Cultivation, Lentiviral Transduction, Generation of a Stable Fluorescent MB49 Cell Line, and Labeling of MB49-GFP Cancer Cells with Metal Nanoparticles

1. Advanced Dulbecco's Modified Eagle Medium /Ham's F-12 (A-DMEM/F-12 (1:1): 0.055 g/L sodium pyruvate, 3.15 g/ L D-glucose, $NaHCO_3$, 15 mM HEPES, phenol red.
2. Reporter gene lentivirus (*see* **Note 1**).
3. Target cells: Mouse bladder carcinoma cell line MB49 (used to induce bladder tumors by intravesical instillation).
4. Dulbecco's Modified Eagle Medium (DMEM) +10% FBS + 1% Penicillin/Streptomycin Solution.
5. Selection antibiotic puromycin (*see* **Notes 1, 10**).
6. Cobalt ferrite nanoparticles ($CoFe_2O_4$).
7. Trypsin.
8. Trypan Blue stain.
9. Cell culture flasks.
10. 6-well plate.
11. 96-well plate (*see* **Note 2**).
12. Serological pipettes.
13. Hemocytometer or cell counter.
14. CO_2 incubator.
15. Laminar flow hood.
16. Fluorescent microscope.

2.2 Materials for Animal Model

Young adult female C57BL/6JOLaHsd mice should be kept in open-bar cages (2–5 per cage) with bedding and enrichment material (paper towel, mouse house) under controlled conditions of temperature (22 ± 1 °C), humidity (55 ± 10%), and light (12 h/12 h light–dark cycle with light from 7 am to 7 pm) with unlimited access to food (standard rodent diet) and water (*see* **Note 3**). Animals should be monitored daily for body weight and behavior throughout the experiment. For long-term experiments, animals should be monitored daily for clinical conditions and for hematuria by palpation of the urinary bladder or by observation of blood on bedding and white paper towel (enrichment material), and weekly for food and water consumed. If there is a loss of more than 20% of body weight, gross hematuria, or signs of pain, premature euthanasia should be performed by the humane endpoint protocol, which is consistent with the principles of the 3Rs for more humane animal research.

1. Phosphate-buffered saline (PBS): pH 7.2–7.4. For stock solution (20×) weigh 4 g KN_2PO_4, 23 g Na_2HPO_4, 4 g KCl, and 160 g NaCl and add 810 mL distilled water. For working solution mix 100 mL of stock solution with 1900 mL distilled water.
2. Anesthetic: 100 mg/kg ketamine HCl and 10 mg/kg xylazine.
3. Pretreatment solution for urothelial injury with 0.01% dispersion of poly-L-lysine hydrobromide (PLL): pH 6.5. Weigh 0.01 g PLL (molecular weight 70–150 kDa) and dissolve in a phosphate buffer.
4. Fine surgical tools for animal research.
5. Animal boards.
6. Micropore medical tape.
7. Polyethylene catheter with an inner diameter of 0.28 mM.
8. 30 G needle connected to a 1 mL injection.
9. Euthanasia chamber for mice.
10. 3% paraformaldehyde in PBS: Dissolve 3 g paraformaldehyde in 100 mL PBS working solution.
11. 10% neutral buffered formalin: Mix 100 mL 37–40% formaldehyde, 900 mL distilled water, 4 g NaH_2PO_4 and 6.5 g Na_2HPO_4 until dissolved.
12. 70% ethanol, 90% ethanol, and 100% ethanol.
13. Xylene.
14. Paraffin embedding molds.
15. Microscope slides and coverslips.
16. Tissue freezing medium.
17. Hematoxylin and eosin stains.

18. Mounting medium with DAPI.
19. Primary and secondary antibodies of interest.
20. 0.4% Triton X-100 in PBS.
21. 3% Bovine serum albumin in PBS.
22. 0.2 M cacodylate buffer: pH 7.3. Mix 62.5 mL Na cacodylate, 3.37 mL 0.2 M HCl, and add distilled water to 250 mL.
23. Fixative solution for transmission electron microscopy (TEM): mixture of 4% paraformaldehyde and 2% glutaraldehyde in 0.2 M cacodylate buffer (pH 7.3). Dissolve 1.15 g paraformaldehyde in 12.5 mL distilled water at 70 °C for 10 min with constant mixing. Add 1 N NaOH dropwise until the solution becomes clear. Cool to room temperature. Add 12.5 mL 0.2 M cacodylate buffer. Immediately prior use add 2 mL 2% glutaraldehyde.
24. Rinsing solution for TEM: 0.33 M sucrose in 0.1 M cacodylate buffer. Mix 11.3 g sucrose, 50 mL 0.2 M cacodylate buffer, and 50 mL distilled water.
25. Secondary fixative solution for transmission electron microscopy (TEM): prepare 1% OsO_4 in 0.2 M cacodylate buffer (pH 7.3) from a 2% aqueous solution of OsO_4.
26. Fixative solution for scanning electron microscope (SEM): mixture of 2% paraformaldehyde and 2% glutaraldehyde in 0.1 M cacodylate buffer (pH 7.4). Dissolve 0.5 g paraformaldehyde in 12.5 mL distilled water at 70 °C for 10 min with constant mixing. Add 1 N NaOH dropwise until the solution becomes clear. Cool to room temperature. Add 12.5 mL of 0.2 M cacodylate buffer. Immediately before use, add 2 mL 2% glutaraldehyde.
27. Toluidine blue stain for semithin sections: dissolve 1 g toluidine blue and 1 g sodium tetraborate (borax) in 100 mL distilled water.
28. Uranyl acetate as staining solution for TEM: for the stock solution of uranyl acetate dissolve 7 g of uranyl acetate in 30 mL of distilled water. The solution should be stored in the dark at room temperature. Filter it through a syringe filter immediately before use. Be careful, the solution is radioactive.
29. Lead citrate as staining solution for TEM: Weigh 0.586 g sodium citrate and 0.443 g of $Pb(NO_3)_2$ and dissolve in 10 mL of distilled water for 1 h at room temperature, then add 2.66 mL of 1 N NaOH while stirring. Filter it through a syringe filter and store the solution in insulin syringes at room temperature for up to 1 month.
30. Epon epoxy resin.
31. Conductive silver paste for scanning electron microscopy.

32. Microtome, cryostat, and ultramicrotome.
33. Critical point dryer.
34. Sputter coater.
35. Bright-field microscope.
36. Fluorescence microscope.
37. Transmission electron microscope (TEM).
38. Scanning electron microscope (SEM).

3 Methods

3.1 Preparation of Fluorescent Monoclonal Stable Cancer Cell Line MB49-GFP Using Lentiviral Transduction (See Note 4)

The first part of the protocol describes the generation of a polyclonal cell culture expressing a fluorescent reporter gene from an integrated lentiviral vector, and the second part of the protocol describes the generation of a monoclonal cell line from a polyclonal population of stably transduced cells by dilutional cloning (*see* **Note 5**).

1. A day before the transduction, plate your target cells in a 6-well plate in 2 mL of DMEM complete media and incubate at 37 ° C, 5% CO_2 overnight (*see* **Note 6**).
2. Next day, aspirate the medium from the cells. Add lentivirus in 2 mL of DMEM (*see* **Note 7**). Mix gently to ensure contact between virus and cells. Incubate at 37 °C, 5% CO_2 overnight.
3. Next day, remove the virus-containing media and rinse the cells twice with 2 mL of PBS. Add 2 mL of fresh DMEM complete media (*see* **Note 8**). Incubate at 37 °C, 5% CO_2 overnight.
4. Next day, you can check the transduced cells under a fluorescence microscope (*see* **Note 9**).
5. Replace the media with 2 mL of DMEM complete media with the selection antibiotic. The well with untransduced cells can be used as a positive control for the antibiotic selection (*see* **Note 10**).
6. In the following 14 days, change to fresh selection antibiotic-containing media every 3–5 days and passage the cells if necessary (*see* **Note 11**).
7. For the selection of monoclonal cell line, trypsinize the polyclonal population and prepare a single-cell suspension by passing the suspension several times through a serological pipette. Determine the cell concentration with a hemocytometer or cell counter (*see* **Note 12**).
8. Transfer cells from the homogenized cell solution into the fresh complete medium to make a new cell solution at a concentration of 1 cell/100 μL or 10 cells/mL. Prepare approximately 10 mL of cell solution to plate a 96-well plate (*see* **Note 13**).

9. Transfer 100 μL of the suspension into each well of a 96-well plate to plate the cells at an average density of 1 cells/well (*see* **Note 14**).
10. Leave the cells undisturbed in an incubator for 7–14 days (*see* **Note 15**).
11. When cells start to form colonies, scan the entire plate and make note of each well in which you detect growing colonies.
12. Select the wells that contain only one colony and pick the population that has the most desirable level of expression.
13. Expend the cells in the selected well by plating them into a larger culture dish. Once the monoclonal lines have been sufficiently expanded, you can prepare a frozen cell stock.

3.2 In Vitro Labeling of MB49-GFP Cancer Cells with Metal Nanoparticles

1. The day before intravesical instillation into animals, expose MB49-GFP cancer cells (*see* **Note 16**) to metal nanoparticles (e.g., $CoFe_2O_4$) at a concentration of 100 μg/mL for 24 h.
2. After incubation with the metal nanoparticles, wash the cells with fresh cell culture medium.
3. Check the viability of the cells with a trypan blue assay.
4. Prepare a single cell suspension of MB49-GFP cancer cells and resuspend them in A-DMEM/F12 (1:1) medium before injecting into animals.

3.3 Establishment of Orthotopic Bladder Tumor Model

1. Anesthetize the mice with an intraperitoneal injection of 100 mg/kg ketamine HCl and 10 mg/kg xylazine and watch for signs of deep anesthesia.
2. Place the mice in the dorsal position and immobilize them by Micropore medical tape on the surgical board.
3. Insert a polyethylene catheter with an inner diameter of 0.28 mM through the vulva and urethra into the urinary bladder (*see* **Note 17**).
4. Once the catheter is inserted into the bladder, carefully insert a 30 G needle connected to a 1 mL syringe into the catheter (*see* **Note 18**).
5. Empty the animal's bladder by applying gentle manual pressure to the lower abdomen.
6. Pretreat the urinary bladder by slowly injecting a volume of 80 μL of a 0.01% dispersion of poly-L-lysine hydrobromide solution with a molecular weight of 70–150 kDa (*see* **Note 19**).
7. After 20 min, gently press on the animal's lower abdomen with a finger to push the poly-L-lysine out of the bladder.
8. Flush poly-L-lysine from the bladder by slowly injecting A-DMEM/F12 medium into the bladder via a catheter.

9. Finally, slowly inject 3×10^6 metal nanoparticle-labeled MB49-GFP cancer cells suspended in 80 μL of A-DMEM/F12 medium into the bladder via a catheter and let the solution in the bladder for 45–60 min. The catheter should be held in place in the meantime to avoid emptying the bladder (*see* **Note 20**).
10. Carefully remove the syringe from the catheter and then slowly withdraw the catheter from the bladder.

3.4 Euthanasia of Animals

1. You should classify the animals into four groups according to the incubation period of the cancer cells in the urinary bladder. Sacrifice group I animals 2 h after the intravesical injection of the cancer cells, group II animals 1 day after the intravesical injection of the cancer cells, group III animals 3 days after the intravesical injection of the cancer cells, and group IV animals 21 days after the intravesical injection of the cancer cells.
2. Perform euthanasia of the animals at the endpoint of each experiment by CO_2 inhalation in the euthanasia chamber (Fig. 2).

3.5 Preparation of Whole-Mount Bladder Tissue Samples

1. Excise the urinary bladders from animals, cut the excised urinary bladder into small flat pieces, and fix them in 3% paraformaldehyde in phosphate-buffered saline (PBS) for 2 h (*see* **Note 21**).
2. Rinse the tissue pieces in PBS.

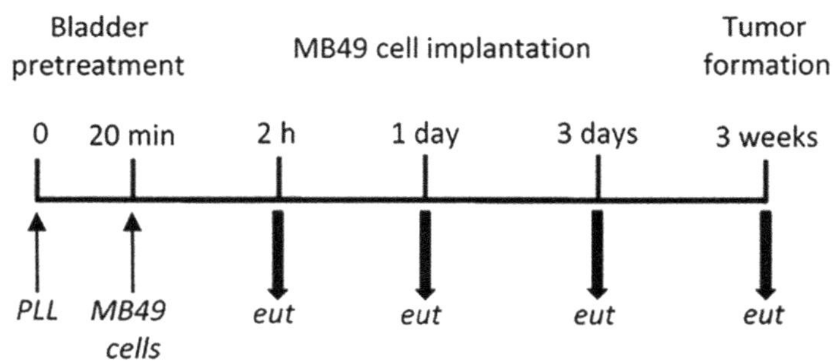

Fig. 2 Schematic overview of the experimental setup and euthanasia plan (eut). The thin arrows show the insertion of the catheter and the thick arrows the time of euthanasia of the animals and tissue sampling. The urothelium was pretreated by intravesical injection of poly-L-lysine (PLL) for 20 min. Subsequently, MB49-GFP cancer cells labeled with metal nanoparticles were introduced into the bladder lumen, and the animals were sacrificed after 2 h, 1 day, 3 days, and 3 weeks. Short-term experiments (2 h, 1 day, and 3 days) are required for the detection of cancer cells, while long-term experiments (3 weeks) are required for tumor analysis

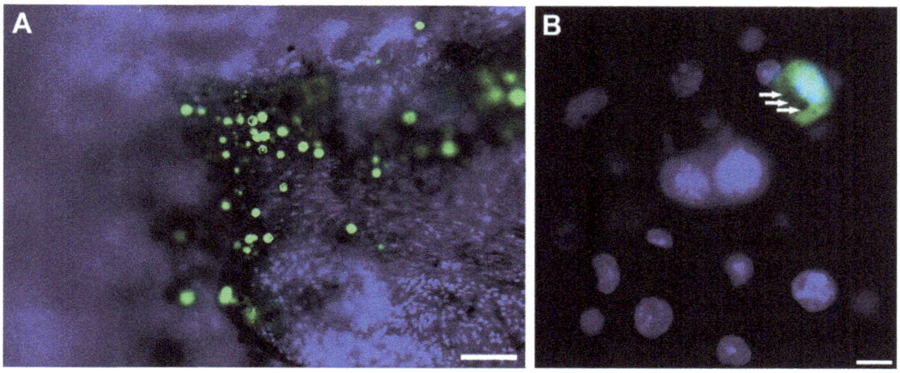

Fig. 3 (**a**) Bird's eye view of attached MB49-GFP cancer cells (green fluorescence by GFP) on the luminal surface of the urinary bladder 3 h after intravesical application of cancer cells in a mouse. (**b**) Higher magnification of MB49-GFP cancer cell (green fluorescence) attached to the luminal surface of the urinary bladder. Dark spots without green fluorescence (arrows) in cytoplasm represent internalized metal nanoparticles in endosomes. Nuclei are stained with DAPI (blue fluorescence). Scale bars: 50 μm (**a**), 10 μm (**b**)

3. Place the tissue pieces luminal side up in a drop of PBS or fluorescence mounting medium on the microscope slide and cover with the cover glass (*see* **Note 22**).
4. Observe the attached MB49-GFP cancer cells on the luminal surface of the urinary bladder wall using a fluorescence or confocal microscope (Fig. 3a, b).

3.6 Observation of Bladder Tumor Growth with the Stereomicroscope

1. Remove the animal's urinary bladder and carefully cut it in half so as not to damage developed tumors in the bladder.
2. Observe the developed tumors on the luminal side of the bladder, either fresh incubated in phosphate buffered saline (PBS) or fixed with 10% neutral buffered formalin (Fig. 4).

3.7 Preparation of Paraffin Sections of Tumor Tissue (for Long-Term Experiments)

1. Cut the excised urinary bladder in half and fix in 10% neutral buffered formalin for 24 h at 4 °C.
2. Dehydrate the tissue pieces in a rising ethanol series and in xylene and embed them in paraffin for 24 h (change the paraffin in the meantime).
3. Cut 4–5 μm thick paraffin sections using the microtome.
4. Deparaffinize the tissue sections in xylene, rehydrate them in decreasing concentrations of ethanol and stain with hematoxylin and eosin (H&E staining).
5. Dehydrate the tissue sections in a rising ethanol series, immerse in xylene, mount in a drop of mounting fluid and cover with coverslips to prepare permanent slides.
6. Observe the developed tumors on the prepared slides using a bright-field microscope (Fig. 5).

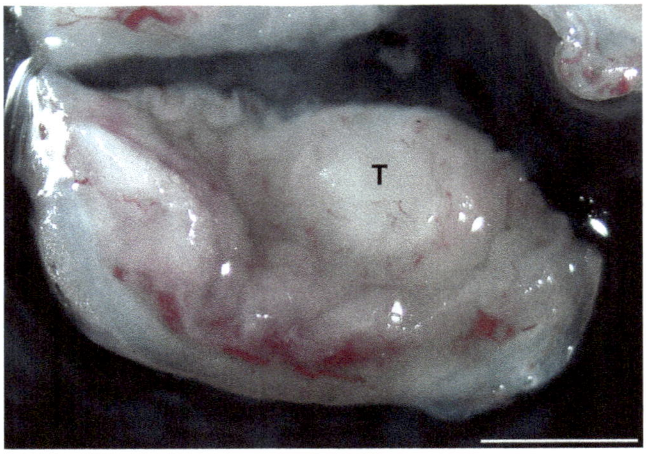

Fig. 4 A piece of fresh bladder tissue with tumor formation (T) 3 weeks after intravesical application of cancer cells in a mouse. Scale bar: 500 μm

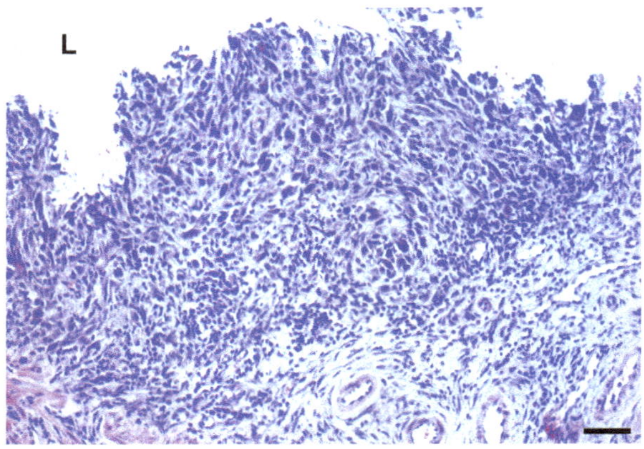

Fig. 5 Histological section of bladder tissue with tumor formation observed 3 weeks after intravesical application of cancer cells in a mouse. Hematoxylin and eosin staining of the paraffin section. L-lumen of the urinary bladder. Scale bar: 100 μm

3.8 Preparation of Cryosections of Bladder Tissue for Fluorescence Microscopy Analysis (for Short- and Long-Term Experiments)

1. Cut the excised urinary bladder in half and fix in 3% paraformaldehyde in PBS for 2 h at 4 °C.
2. Incubate the tissue pieces overnight with 30% sucrose at 4 °C.
3. The next day, embed the tissue pieces in tissue freezing medium, freeze them in the cryostat chamber at −30 °C and cut 4–5 μm thick cryosections on the cryostat.
4. Use the prepared cryosections to perform labeling of cell nuclei with DAPI by mounting the cryosections in the mounting medium with DAPI.

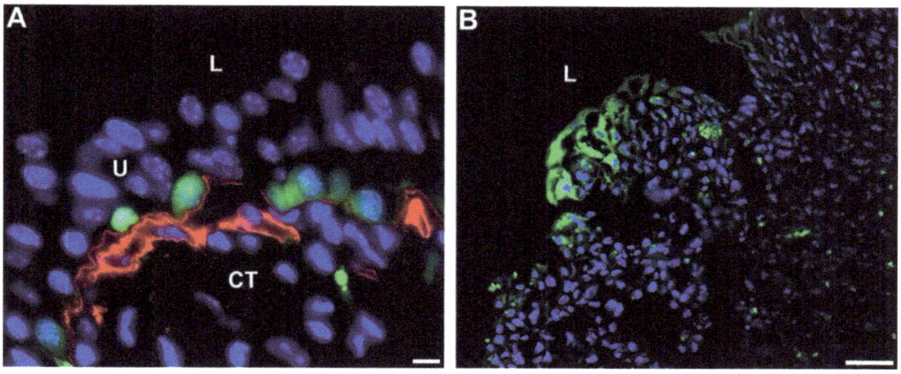

Fig. 6 Cryosections with implanted MB49-GFP cancer cells (green fluorescence by GFP) within the urothelium reaching the underlying basal lamina (red fluorescence by immunofluorescence labeling of collagen IV) 3 days after intravesical application of cancer cells in a mouse (**a**) and tumor formation (green fluorescence by GFP) 3 weeks after intravesical application of cancer cells in a mouse (**b**). L-lumen of the urinary bladder, U-urothelium, CT-connective tissue. Scale bars: 100 μm

5. Optionally, perform immunolabeling (immunofluorescence) with antibodies for cancer cell-specific antigens or any histological component of interest: permeabilize the tissue samples (e.g., with 0.4% Triton X-100 in PBS for 5 min), incubate tissue specimens in a blocking solution (e.g., 3% bovine serum albumin in PBS for 1 h), then incubate overnight with selected primary antibodies and later with appropriate fluorophore-conjugated secondary antibodies (1 h), mount in the mounting medium and cover with coverslips.
6. Observe MB49-GFP cancer cells bound to the urothelium or implanted in the bladder wall using a fluorescence microscope (Fig. 6).

3.9 Preparation of Semithin and Ultrathin Sections of Bladder Tissue for Transmission Electron Microscopy (TEM) Analysis

1. Cut the excised urinary bladder into small pieces (*see* **Note 23**).
2. Fix the bladder pieces in a mixture of 4% paraformaldehyde and 2% glutaraldehyde in 0.2 M cacodylate buffer (pH 7.3) for 3 h at 4 °C (*see* **Note 24**).
3. Incubate the tissue pieces overnight with 0.33 M sucrose in 0.2 M cacodylate buffer.
4. The next day, perform postfixation with 1% OsO_4 for 1 h.
5. Dehydrate the tissue pieces in an increasing ethanol series.
6. Embed the tissue samples in epoxy resin Epon.
7. Cut Epon semithin sections (1 μm thick) on the ultramicrotome and stain them for 20 s with toluidine blue and observe them with a bright-field microscope (*see* **Note 25**).
8. Cut 50 nM thick ultrathin sections with the ultramicrotome and contrast them with uranyl acetate and lead citrate.

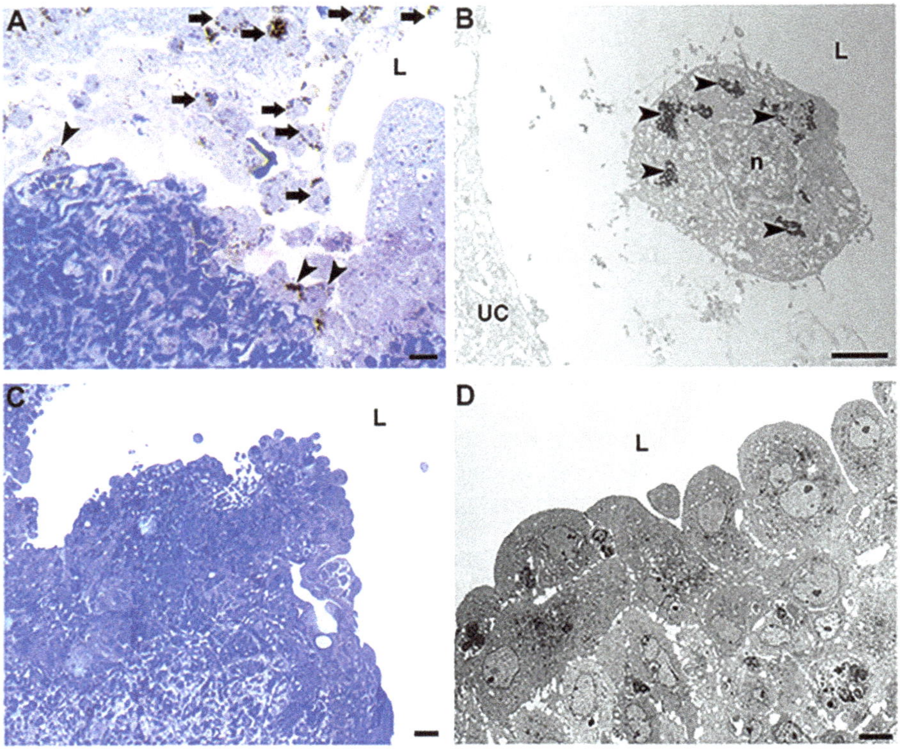

Fig. 7 Semithin and ultrathin sections of injected MB49 cancer cells in the urinary bladder lumen 2 h after intravesical application (**a**, **b**) and tumors 3 weeks after intravesical application of cancer cells in a mouse (**c**, **d**). (**a**) Semithin section of numerous cancer cells labeled with metal nanoparticles (arrows) floating in the bladder lumen and three cancer cells already attached to the urothelium or exposed basal lamina (arrowheads). (**b**) Ultrathin section of a cancer cell labeled with metal nanoparticles (arrowheads) in the lumen of the urinary bladder and in close proximity to the urothelial cell (UC). (**c**) Semithin section of the tumor formation. (**d**) Ultrathin section of tumor cells as part of tumor formation. L-lumen of the urinary bladder, n-nucleus. Scale bars: 10 μm (**a**), 2 μm (b), 50 μm (**c**), 10 μm (**d**)

9. View semithin sections with a bright-field microscope (Fig. 7a, c) and ultrathin sections with a transmission electron microscope (Fig. 7b, d).

3.10 Preparation of Bladder Tissue Specimens for Scanning Electron Microscopy (SEM) Analysis

1. Remove the urinary bladder of the animal (*see* **Note 26**).
2. Cut the urinary bladder in half lengthwise and fix in a mixture of 2% paraformaldehyde and 2% glutaraldehyde in 0.1 M cacodylate buffer (pH 7.4) for 3–4 h at 4 °C.
3. Rinse the tissue samples in 0.1 M cacodylate buffer and then fix them in 1% OsO_4 in the same buffer for 1 h at 4 °C.
4. Dry the samples in a critical point dryer.
5. Mount the samples on brass or aluminum holders with conductive silver paste.

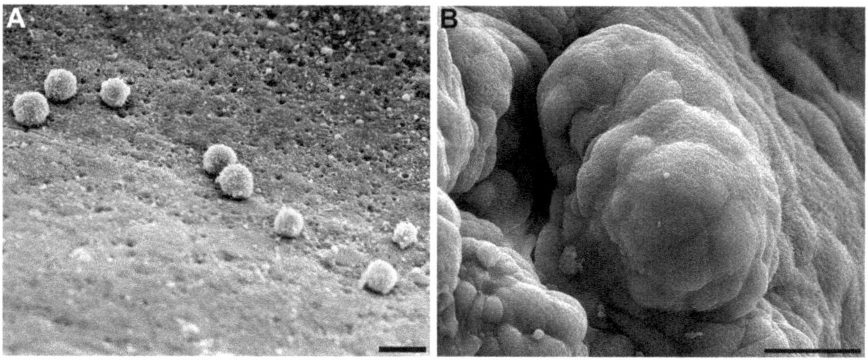

Fig. 8 Scanning electron micrographs of cancer cells attached to the luminal surface of the urothelium 2 h after intravesical application of cancer cells in a mouse (**a**) and bladder tumor formation 3 weeks after intravesical application of cancer cells in a mouse (**b**). Scale bars: 10 μm (**a**), 50 μm (**b**)

6. Coat the samples with gold in the sputter coater.
7. Observe the specimens with the scanning electron microscope (Fig. 8a, b).

4 Notes

1. Premade or custom-made ready-to-use lentiviral particles can be acquired from different providers. Or you can prepare your own particles by transfecting a packaging cell line with packaging plasmids and your target plasmid encoding the selected gene you wish to transduce. For the generation of the MB49-GFP cell line, lentiviral particles were prepared using a third-generation lentiviral system transfected with lipid-based transfection system, such as Lipofectamine 2000 into 293 T cells. The plasmids used were: pLenti PGK GFP Puro transfer plasmid encoding an enhanced green fluorescent protein (eGFP) and the puromycin resistance gene for selection of transduced cells, the packaging plasmids pMDLg/pRRE and pMD2.G, and the envelope plasmid pRSV-Rev.
2. We recommend using black 96-well plates with clear bottoms to reduce well-to-well crosstalk in fluorescence microscopy.
3. We have found that it is useful to deprive the animals of water a few hours before the instillation of the cancer cells into the animals. The animals urinate less frequently, so fewer cancer cells are flushed from the urinary bladder and the growth rate of the tumor is higher.
4. Lentivirus is a modified HIV virus and is considered biosafety level 2 (BSL-2) material. Contact your institution's biosafety office before beginning work with lentivirus.

5. This protocol can be used for cells that can form discrete monoclonal colonies from individual cells.
6. On the day of transduction, cells should be 70% confluent. To minimize the risks associated with lentivirus, use only 1–3 wells for transduction. The rest can be used as nontransduced control and for testing the concentrations of the selection antibiotic (*see* step 5).
7. The most effective amount of virus particles to be added depends on the multiplicity of infection (MOI) and should be determined empirically for each cell line. To increase the efficiency of lentivirus integration, polybrene can be added to the transduction medium at a concentration of 8–10 μg/mL. For the generation of the MB49-GFP cell line, 2 mL of fresh viral supernatant in DMEM was successfully used without the addition of polybrene.
8. The selection antibiotic should not be added before 24 h after transduction to allow sufficient expression of the antibiotic resistance gene.
9. At this stage, the transduced cells should already start to fluoresce.
10. The concentration of puromycin depends on the cell type and can usually be found in the literature or on various websites. However, we recommend determining the optimal dose of antibiotic for your target cell line prior to transduction by treating the target cell with a series of doses of the antibiotic. The lowest dose that kills all cells should be chosen for selection. For the generation of the MB49-GFP cell line, 3 μg/mL puromycin was used.
11. Observe the cells carefully during this time. If the cells become confluent, expand them into larger cell culture flasks. Continue the antibiotic challenge until the uninfected control cells are completely dead. You now have a polyclonal population of resistant cells in which the reporter gene has been inserted at different locations in the genome and at different copy numbers. This can result in differential expression of the transgene in different cells in the population. Over time, the expression of the transgene may decrease in a polyclonal population. Therefore, the generation of a monoclonal cell line is recommended.
12. Prepare a relatively diluted cell solution ($<10^6$ cells/mL) before counting as you will need to prepare a highly diluted cell suspension in the next step.
13. To transfer larger and thus more accurate volumes, prepare 1 mL of a 1:100 dilution of the homogenized cell solution.
14. Fill one of the corner wells of the plate with about 1000 cells so that you can focus the microscope later when you scan the plate for single cells, which can be difficult to find.

15. During this time scan the plate for cell growth.
16. We use the fifth to seventh passage of MB49 cancer cell culture for intravesical instillation.
17. Cut a 4 cm piece from a catheter. Before insertion, mark the catheter with an alcohol marker 0.5 cm, 1 cm, and 1.5 cm from the end to be inserted into the bladder. Then carefully lift the skin of the mouse near the vulva with straight fine forceps to align the urethra, and slowly insert the catheter into the urethra with curved fine forceps. When the catheter is inserted to the third mark (1.5 cm), you can be sure that the catheter is in the bladder.
18. It is important to check that the catheter is in the bladder before inserting the syringe into the catheter. To do this, apply gentle manual pressure to the lower abdomen. If urine comes out of the end of the catheter, you can be sure that it is in the correct position.
19. We recommend using a 0.1 mg/mL poly-L-lysine hydrobromide (PLL) solution with a molecular weight of 70–150 kDa because PLL at this concentration and molecular weight causes massive but safe desquamation of epithelial cells without deeply injuring the bladder epithelium.
20. All injections should be performed gradually and slowly to avoid tissue injury or vesicoureteral reflux.
21. We recommend ligating the urinary bladder with a suture before opening the animal and carefully dilating the bladder by slowly injecting a fixative solution (3% paraformaldehyde in phosphate-buffered saline) to obtain flat pieces of the bladder wall after incision and cutting.
22. If the tissue pieces are thick, we suggest making a small tissue chamber on the microscope slide with silicone paste. Then place the tissue pieces in it with the luminal side up, cover them with the cover glass, and press gently. Another way to create a tissue chamber is to place a dental modeling wax sheet on the microscope slide, make a small hole, fill it with PBS or a fluorescence mounting medium, place the tissue piece in with the luminal side up, cover it with the cover glass, and gently press on.
23. Cut the urinary bladder tissue into 1 mM^3 or smaller pieces to allow better penetration of the fixative.
24. For faster and better fixation of the bladder tissue, we recommend reinserting the catheter into the bladder and injecting the fixative solution through the catheter before urinary bladder removal.

25. It is a common practice to make semithin sections prior to making ultrathin sections so that the region of interest in the tissue can be properly determined for subsequent cutting of ultrathin sections.
26. We have found that the analysis with SEM is easier and better if we ligate the filled and distended urinary bladder with a suture before excising from the animal. The ligated and excised bladder is then quickly placed in the fixative solution and cut in half.

References

1. Gengenbacher N, Singhal M, Augustin HG (2017) Preclinical mouse solid tumour models: status quo, challenges and perspectives. Nat Rev Cancer 17:751–765. https://doi.org/10.1038/nrc.2017.92
2. Zhang N, Li D, Shao J, Wang X (2015) Animal models for bladder cancer: the model establishment and evaluation (review). Oncol Lett 9: 1515–1519. https://doi.org/10.3892/ol.2015.2888
3. Gunther JH (1999) Optimizing syngeneic orthotopic murine bladder cancer(MB49). Cancer Res 59(12):2834–2837
4. Fabris VT, Lodillinsky C, Pampena MB et al (2012) Cytogenetic characterization of the murine bladder cancer model MB49 and the derived invasive line MB49-I. Cancer Genet 205:168–176. https://doi.org/10.1016/j.cancergen.2012.02.002
5. Wu Q (2003) Nonviral cytokine gene therapy on an orthotopic bladder cancer model. Clin Cancer Res 9(12):4522–4528
6. Zaharoff DA, Hoffman BS, Hooper HB et al (2009) Intravesical immunotherapy of superficial bladder cancer with chitosan/Interleukin-12. Cancer Res 69:6192–6199. https://doi.org/10.1158/0008-5472.CAN-09-1114
7. Summerhays (1979) Effects of donor age on neoplastic transformation of adult mouse bladder epithelium in vitro. J Natl Cancer Inst 62(4):1017–1023
8. Erman A, Kapun G, Novak S et al (2019) How cancer cells attach to urinary bladder epithelium in vivo: study of the early stages of tumorigenesis in an orthotopic mouse bladder tumor model. Histochem Cell Biol 151:263–273. https://doi.org/10.1007/s00418-018-1738-x
9. Erman A, Kamenšek U, Dragin Jerman U et al (2021) How cancer cells invade bladder epithelium and form tumors: the mouse bladder tumor model as a model of tumor recurrence in patients. Int J Mol Sci 22:6328. https://doi.org/10.3390/ijms22126328
10. Soloway MS, Masters S (1980) Urothelial susceptibility to tumor cell implantation influence of cauterization. Cancer 46:1158–1163. https://doi.org/10.1002/1097-0142(19800901)46:5<1158::AID-CNCR2820460514>3.0.CO;2-E
11. Loskog A, Ninalga C, Hedlund T et al (2005) Optimization of the MB49 mouse bladder cancer model for adenoviral gene therapy. Lab Anim 39:384–393. https://doi.org/10.1258/002367705774286475
12. Chan E, Patel A, Heston W, Larchian W (2009) Mouse orthotopic models for bladder cancer research. BJU Int 104:1286–1291. https://doi.org/10.1111/j.1464-410X.2009.08577.x
13. Chan ESY, Patel AR, Smith AK et al (2009) Optimizing orthotopic bladder tumor implantation in a syngeneic mouse model. J Urol 182: 2926–2931. https://doi.org/10.1016/j.juro.2009.08.020
14. Soloway MS, Nissenkorn I, McCallum L (1983) Urothelial susceptibility to tumor cell implantation: comparison of cauterization with N-methyl-N-nitrosourea. Urology 21:159–161. https://doi.org/10.1016/0090-4295(83)90013-4
15. Chin J, Kadhim S, Garcia B et al (1991) Magnetic resonance imaging for detecting and treatment monitoring of orthotopic murine bladder tumor implants. J Urol 145:1297–1301. https://doi.org/10.1016/S0022-5347(17)38618-4
16. Werthman PE (1996) Adenoviral-p53 fene transfer to orthotopic and peritoneal murine bladder. J Urol 155(2):753–756
17. Watanabe T, Shinohara N, Sazawa A et al (2000) An improved intravesical model using human bladder cancer cell lines to optimize gene and other therapies. Cancer Gene Ther 7:1575–1580. https://doi.org/10.1038/sj.cgt.7700261

18. Bisson J-F, Parache RM, Droulle P et al (2002) A new method of implanting orthotopic rat bladder tumor for experimental therapies. Int J Cancer 102:280–285. https://doi.org/10.1002/ijc.10595
19. Chade DC, Andrade PM, Borra RC et al (2008) Histopathological characterization of a syngeneic orthotopic murine bladder cancer model. Int Braz J Urol 34:220–229. https://doi.org/10.1590/S1677-55382008000200013
20. Mangsbo SM, Ninalga C, Essand M et al (2008) CpG therapy is superior to BCG in an orthotopic bladder cancer model and generates CD4+ T-cell immunity. J Immunother 31:34–42. https://doi.org/10.1097/CJI.0b013e3181587d29
21. Kerec Kos M, Veranič P, Erman A (2019) Poly-L-lysine as an effective and safe desquamation inducer of urinary bladder epithelium. Polymers 11:1506. https://doi.org/10.3390/polym11091506

Chapter 5

Azoxymethane/Dextran Sodium Sulfate (AOM/DSS) Model of Colorectal Cancer

Mariangela De Robertis and Emanuela Signori

Abstract

Recent progress in developing new vaccination strategies against cancer requires the production of complex and reliable animal models reflecting the complexity of the tumors with their microenvironment. Mice can be considered a good source due to low cost and ease of being genetically modified, inoculated with tumor cell lines or treated by chemicals to induce different cancers. Despite significant limitations in modeling human cancer complexity, preclinical trials conducted in mice can efficiently contribute to understand molecular mechanisms of cancer, to closely resemble and follow carcinogenesis steps impossible to study into humans, and to test new anticancer therapies. In this chapter, we generally describe the different mouse models developed for cancer vaccines' preclinical trials. A particular focus is dedicated to a chemically-induced colorectal cancer model in use in our laboratories.

Key words Mouse models, Cancer vaccines, Colorectal cancer, Chemically-induced tumors, AOM/DSS mouse model

1 Introduction

Vaccines in various forms, such as protein-, nucleic acids-, and cell-based, are now the frontier of oncology research. Cancer vaccines research is focused largely on the development of new therapies that harness the power of the immune system to fight tumors. Mechanistically, cancer vaccines target tumor-associated antigens to enhance the immune response, through an autoimmune function to kill tumor cells, and provide antitumor effects [1].

Among the different treatment modalities in cancer immunotherapy, tumor vaccines have been extensively tested in animal models in the past few decades. In fact, to predict human response to cancer vaccines, candidate formulations should be investigated in a fully functional immune system and only animals carrying an intact immune system can mimic human responses to immune

Maja Čemažar, Tanja Jesenko and Urša Lampreht Tratar (eds.), *Mouse Models of Cancer: Methods and Protocols*, Methods in Molecular Biology, vol. 2773, https://doi.org/10.1007/978-1-0716-3714-2_5,
© The Author(s), under exclusive license to Springer Science+Business Media, LLC, part of Springer Nature 2024

modulation associated to vaccination. Therefore, the choice of animal models is critical in cancer vaccine research.

Different tumor mouse models have been generated as tools for investigating cancer vaccination strategies: (a) genetically engineered mouse models, (b) syngeneic and xenograft models, and (c) chemically-induced models.

Genetically engineered mouse models (GEMMs) can reproduce tumor development, starting from initiated (mutated) cells to cover tumor growth and progression and, potentially, metastases [2]. To date, different mouse models with inducible overexpression or knockout of gene(s), such as c-myc [3], k-ras [4], or Apc [5], have been developed. For example, mutant mice carrying a heterozygous germline mutation in the APC gene (Min/ΔAPC-mouse) develop multiple intestinal neoplasia and mimic the rapid tumor formation seen in familial adenomatous polyposis (FAP) patients [6]. In GEMMs, the evolution of a native tumor microenvironment can be preserved, because tumors are allowed to spontaneously develop in an immunocompetent host. This is crucial as the tumor microenvironment has a great impact on immunotherapies [7]. Although GEMMs have limitations related to the complex development of models capable of accurately recapitulating human diseases, they have recently been used to assess antitumor immune responses after vaccines administration [8].

Syngeneic mouse models are the most frequently used tumor mouse models because they are straightforward and easily achievable and can represent an important step toward a pathobiologically relevant model of tumor metastasis. They are developed by inoculating, via subcutaneous, intraperitoneal, intravenous, or orthotopic injection, in vitro cultured tumor cell lines [9] that are derived from common inbred mouse strains [10]. Maintaining an intact immune system in these syngeneic mouse models allows for immunotherapy evaluation [10, 11]. A recent implementation of another model consists of patient-derived xenografts (PDXs) tumor models, which can be generated by implanting surgically removed tumor fragments from patients into immunocompromised animals. These models allow to transfer the patient malignancy and its tumor microenvironment, to an animal model [12, 13]. However, their deficient intrinsic immune systems make PDX models unsuitable for evaluating immunotherapies. For this reason, the improvement of humanized PDX models with an immune system that is autologous to the implanted tumor [14] or with a human immune system [15] has recently been achieved, making it possible to use such PDX models to evaluate cancer vaccination strategies.

Chemically-induced tumor mouse models are generated by administering a carcinogen to rodents to induce the same stages of tumor initiation and progression that occur in humans. Such models are often used to evaluate the activity of chemopreventive compounds, to identify cancer risk factors, and to test immunotherapeutic strategies. These models can recapitulate different types of human tumors with high reproducibility in animals with different genetic backgrounds. In particular, a variety of chemical agents have been used to induce colon tumors in mice, such as heterocyclic amines, aromatic amines, alkylnitrosamide compounds, and dimethylhydrazine and azoxymethane.

Among them, we used azoxymethane (AOM), an alkylating agent which induces DNA-reactive adducts, combined with the inflammatory agent dextran sodium sulfate (DSS) to obtain a mouse model of inflammation-driven sporadic colorectal cancer (CRC) [16]. We observed that the administration of AOM with DSS in drinking water causes rapid growth of multiple colon tumors per mouse within 10 weeks [16]. In fact, the AOM/DSS combined protocol dramatically shortens the latency time observed in the classical model of spontaneous CRC, which is based on several repeated intraperitoneal (i.p.) AOM injections [17]. AOM/DSS-induced tumors develop with high frequency within the distal colon of mice by a multistep process in which normal crypts are initiated to form foci of aberrant crypts (ACF) that proliferate and evolve through an adenoma–carcinoma sequence [18]. Tumors exhibit histopathological features similar to CRC in man, but often lack mucosal invasiveness, and metastasis is very rare [19]. Importantly, identification of ACF in AOM/DSS-treated mice makes the study of CRC at the precancerous stages possible with this model. Since the total number and size of ACF can be scored easily, the evaluation of these small lesions can be used as a short-term bioassay to evaluate the effect of immunotherapy or chemopreventive agents as well as nutritional components at an early stage of colon carcinogenesis.

Advantages of AOM/DSS-induced CRC mouse model include high potency and reproducibility, simple mode of application, and low price. We exploited the AOM/DSS model to characterize potential new biomarkers of CRC pathogenesis [20–23], some of which could be used to design novel immunotherapeutic strategies. Other investigators also used this model to test cancer vaccines efficacy [24] or different immunotherapeutic approaches [25, 26].

2 Materials

2.1 Mice

Sex-matched mice aged 6–8 weeks of 18–20 g body weight and belonging to a strain of high or moderate susceptibility to AOM, such as Balb/c, C57BL/6, A/J, SWR/J, and FVB/N strains. A minimum of nine animals per group are recommended (*see* **Note 1**).

2.2 AOM Solution

Dilute AOM in sterile isotonic 0.9% NaCl at 0.5 mg/mL (*see* **Note 2**). Prepare this solution in sterile conditions and filter with 0.22 μm membranes. Once the solution is prepared, make aliquots and store them at −20 °C for up to 1 year (*see* **Note 3**).

2.3 DSS Solution

To obtain a 2% (wt/vol) solution, dissolve 2 g of DSS powder per 100 mL filtered water (*see* **Note 4**). Prepare the solution in sterile conditions. Store DSS solution for up to 1 week at 2–8 °C. Calculate the amount needed by allowing 5 mL DSS solution per mouse per day (*see* **Note 5**). Frequency of bottle change: every 2 days.

2.4 Drinking Water

Deliver filtered water in a bottle for each cage ad libitum.

2.5 Additional Materials and Equipment

Anesthesia machine, isoflurane, analytical balance, laminar airflow hood, anatomical forceps and scissors, sterile syringes, Petri dishes, cold PBS.

3 Methods

3.1 Chemical Induction of Tumor Development

1. Distribute animals equally into experimental and control groups to ensure adequate group size (*see* **Note 1**).
2. On day 0, weigh and label the animals with earmarking.
3. Calculate the amount of AOM needed (e.g., 10 mg per kg body weight) and thaw as many aliquots of stock solution as necessary.
4. Prepare AOM solution at a concentration of 0.5 mg/mL and inject intraperitoneally AOM solution (10 mg per kg body weight) for the experimental group or sterile isotonic saline for the control group (*see* **Note 6**).
5. Prepare 2% DSS solution and fill the water bottles of the cages with an adequate volume of DSS-containing water for 3 days (*see* **Note 7**). Change the cage water bottles at day 4 and day 6 and refill with fresh DSS solution for 2 more days, respectively.

   Change the cage water bottles at day 8 and refill with autoclaved water.
6. Evaluate for precursor lesions at weeks 5–6 and for tumor development at weeks 10–12 as in Fig. 1 (*see* **Note 8**) by euthanizing three of the animals from the group and dissecting them for macroscopic inspection of the colon and histological analysis of colon mucosa.

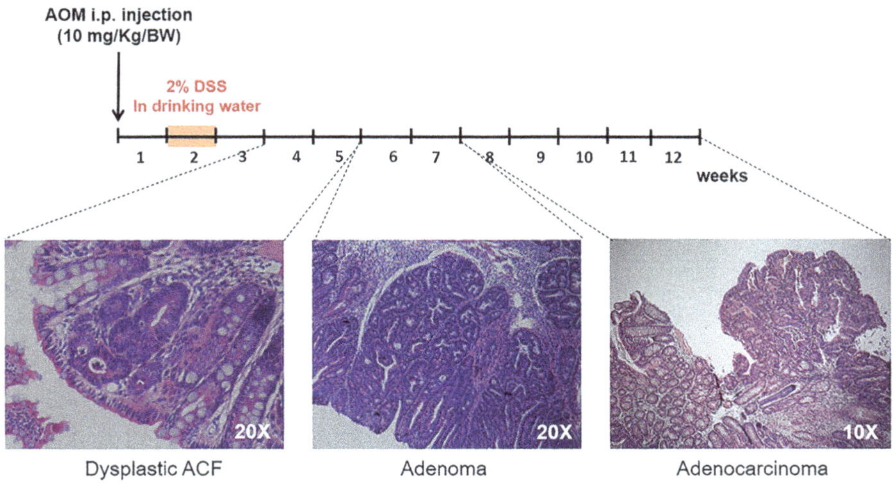

Fig. 1 Scheme of AOM/DSS experimental protocol and timing of multiphase colorectal cancer development in inbred Balb/c mice

3.2 Macroscopic Inspection and Tissue Sampling for the Evaluation of Tumor and Precancerous Lesions

1. Humanely kill the mice by cervical dislocation under anesthesia at the time points of interest (*see* **Note 9**).
2. Surgically open the bowel cavity and carefully remove the colon with anatomical forceps and scissors. Place the colon in a Petri dish filled with cold PBS (*see* **Note 10**).
3. Carefully open the colon longitudinally and rinse with cold PBS to remove residual feces (*see* **Note 11**).
4. Analyze tumor development according to the purpose of the study (Fig. 2): (a) macroscopic quantification of tumor load through assessment of tumor numbers and size (average diameter); (b) detection of ACFs and tumors through standard procedures of histopathological analysis; (c) molecular and/or biochemical analysis on fresh frozen tumors and normal colon tissues.

4 Notes

1. All experiments involving rodents must conform with local and national animal care regulations and adhere to ethical standards.
2. AOM is more stable in water or isotonic saline than in buffered PBS and is more stable in glassware than in plastic tubes.
3. AOM is carcinogenic to humans and is a flammable substance. Hence, when handling AOM, wear protective equipment including gloves and face protection. Injections should be performed by skilled experimenters.

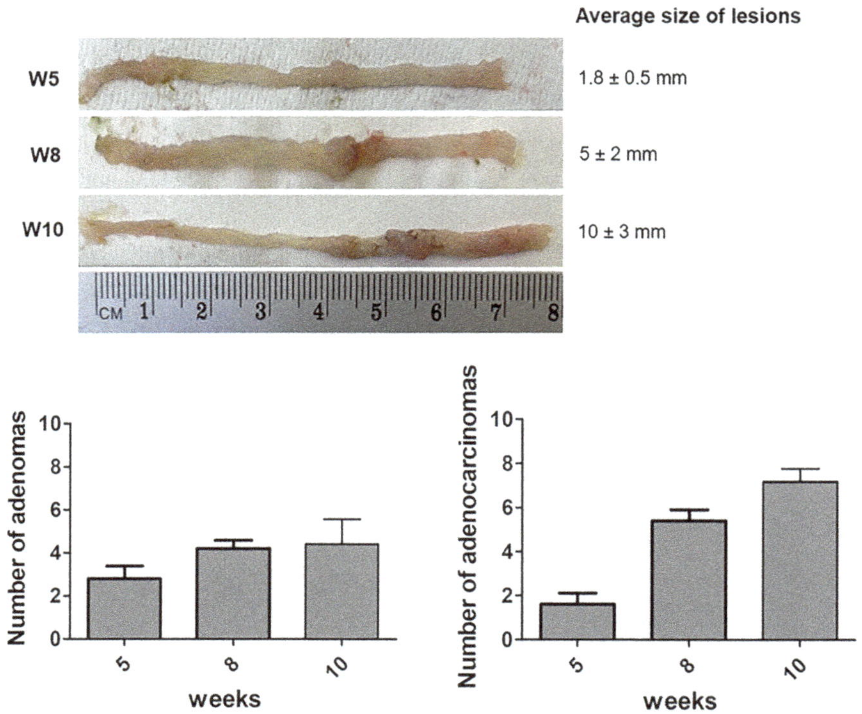

Fig. 2 Macroscopic analysis showing early and late colon neoplasms developed in AOM/DSS-treated mice at 5, 8, and 10 weeks from the start of the AOM/DSS protocol. Tumors are localized exclusively within the distal colon. The number of adenomas and carcinomas per colon is also reported

4. DSS is toxic to mice, ensuing in bloody feces.
5. According to the susceptibility of different mouse strains to DSS-induced colitis, DSS concentration can be decreased or increased between 1% and 3% (wt/vol). Alternatively, the period of DSS administration could be reduced to 4–5 days.
6. Use a sterile syringe in a laminar airflow hood.
7. Make sure the tip of the lids is not engorged.
8. Early lesions such as aberrant crypt foci (ACFs) or mucin-depleted foci (MDFs) represent early end points and should be scored at about 5 weeks while more advanced lesions such as adenomas and adenocarcinomas should be scored at 8 and 10 weeks, respectively.
9. Record any clinical abnormality and treat as appropriate to minimize animal pain and distress. Major abdomen distension and major hematochezia are considered as specific endpoints, and their observation is immediately followed by animals' euthanasia.
10. Make sure not to bruise the colon tissue with the forceps.

11. Make sure not to cut into the tumors, but to cut between them.

Acknowledgments

This work was supported by Project CNR-DSB.AD007.257.

References

1. Parish CR (2003) Cancer immunotherapy: the past, the present and the future. Immunol Cell Biol 81:106–113
2. Van Dyke T, Jacks T (2002) Cancer modeling in the modern era: progress and challenges. Cell 108:135–144
3. Stewart TA, Pattengale PK, Leder P (1984) Spontaneous mammary adenocarcinomas in transgenic mice that carry and express MTV/myc fusion genes. Cell 38:627–637
4. Quaife CJ, Pinkert CA, Ornitz DM et al (1987) Pancreatic neoplasia induced by ras expression in acinar cells of transgenic mice. Cell 48:1023–1034
5. Moser AR, Luongo C, Gould KA et al (1995) ApcMin: a mouse model for intestinal and mammary tumorigenesis. Eur J Cancer 31A:1061–1064
6. Fodde R, Smits R (2001) Disease model: familial adenomatous polyposis. Trends Mol Med 7: 369–373
7. Zhang J, Shi Z, Xu X et al (2019) The influence of microenvironment on tumor immunotherapy. FEBS J 286:4160–4175
8. Arbelaez CA, Estrada J, Gessner MA et al (2020) A nanoparticle vaccine that targets neoantigen peptides to lymphoid tissues elicits robust antitumor T cell responses. NPJ Vaccines 5:106
9. Talmadge JE, Singh RK, Fidler IJ et al (2007) Murine models to evaluate novel and conventional therapeutic strategies for cancer. Am J Pathol 170:793–804
10. DeVita VT Jr, Chu E (2008) A history of cancer chemotherapy. Cancer Res 68:8643–8653
11. Komel T, Bosnjak M, Kranjc Brezar S et al (2021) Gene electrotransfer of IL-2 and IL-12 plasmids effectively eradicated murine B16.F10 melanoma. Bioelectrochemistry 141: 107843
12. Reyal F, Guyader C, Decraene C et al (2012) Molecular profiling of patient-derived breast cancer xenografts. Breast Cancer Res 14:R11
13. Evans KW, Yuca E, Akcakanat A et al (2017) A population of heterogeneous breast cancer patient-derived xenografts demonstrate broad activity of PARP inhibitor in BRCA1/2 wild-type tumors. Clin Cancer Res 23:6468–6477
14. Wang M, Yao L-C, Cheng M et al (2018) Humanized mice in studying efficacy and mechanisms of PD-1-targeted cancer immunotherapy. FASEB J 32:1537–1549
15. Jangalwe S, Shultz LD, Mathew A et al (2016) Improved B cell development in humanized NOD-scid IL2Rγ(null) mice transgenically expressing human stem cell factor, granulocyte-macrophage colony-stimulating factor and interleukin-3. Immun Inflamm Dis 4:427–440
16. De Robertis M, Massi E, Poeta ML et al (2011) The AOM/DSS murine model for the study of colon carcinogenesis: from pathways to diagnosis and therapy studies. J Carcinog 10:9
17. Jackson PE, Cooper DP, O'Connor PJ et al (1999) The relationship between 1,2-dimethylhydrazine dose and the induction of colon tumours: tumour development in female SWR mice does not require a K-ras mutational event. Carcinogenesis 20:509–513
18. Kinzler KW, Vogelstein B (1996) Lessons from hereditary colorectal cancer. Cell 87:159–170
19. Kobaek-Larsen M, Thorup I, Diederichsen A et al (2000) Review of colorectal cancer and its metastases in rodent models: comparative aspects with those in humans. Comp Med 50: 16–26
20. De Robertis M, Arigoni M, Loiacono L et al (2015) Novel insights into Notum and glypicans regulation in colorectal cancer. Oncotarget 6:41237–41257
21. De Robertis M, Greco MR, Cardone RA et al (2022) Upregulation of YKL-40 promotes metastatic phenotype and correlates with poor prognosis and therapy response in patients with colorectal cancer. Cells 11:3568
22. De Robertis M, Loiacono L, Fusilli C et al (2017) Dysregulation of EGFR pathway in EphA2 cell subpopulation significantly

associates with poor prognosis in colorectal cancer. Clin Cancer Res 23:159–170

23. De Robertis M, Mazza T, Fusilli C et al (2018) EphB2 stem-related and EphA2 progression-related miRNA-based networks in progressive stages of CRC evolution: clinical significance and potential miRNA drivers. Mol Cancer 17: 169

24. Singh S, Singh M, Gaur S (2022) Probiotics as multifaceted oral vaccines against colon cancer: a review. Front Immunol 13:1002674

25. Yassin M, Sadowska Z, Djurhuus D et al (2019) Upregulation of PD-1 follows tumour development in the AOM/DSS model of inflammation-induced colorectal cancer in mice. Immunology 158:35–46

26. Zhang X, Wei L, Wang J et al (2017) Suppression colitis and colitis-associated colon cancer by anti-S100a9 antibody in mice. Front Immunol 8:1774

Chapter 6

Isolating Primary Tumor Cells from the MMTV-PyMT Mouse Model and Their Use in Developing an Orthotopic Mouse Model of Breast Cancer

Andreja Kozak, Olga Vasiljeva, and Georgy Mikhaylov

Abstract

To study the effect of the immunologically unimpaired microenvironment on tumor progression as well as the efficacy of therapies requiring a functioning immune system, xenograft models are not suitable due to the use of immunodeficient mice. With orthotopic congenic transplantation of tumor cells into mammary tissue, we gain more control and reproducibility regarding tumor growth, while retaining a functioning immune response. Here, we provide a protocol for isolating primary tumor cells from the MMTV-PyMT mouse model and their use in developing an orthotopic mouse model of breast cancer.

Key words Breast cancer, Mouse model, Mammary adenocarcinoma, Orthotopic transplantation, Polyomavirus middle T antigen

1 Introduction

Breast cancer is one of the leading causes of cancer-related female death worldwide, even though clinical treatment has improved significantly in the last decades. The search for a better understanding of breast cancer pathology and novel or improved therapies has relied heavily on in vivo experimental models of the disease. There are three major types of mouse models of breast cancer based on the tumor development/initiation mechanisms: tumor transplantation models, genetically engineered models, and chemical carcinogenesis models.

Tumor transplantation models include cell-derived xenografts (CDX), patient-derived xenografts (PDX), and syngeneic models. Both CDX and PDX are applied to immunocompromised mice. For the former, human cancer cell lines are used to transplant tumors subcutaneously, while for PDX models, primary human breast carcinomas or tumor fragments are used. The main advantages of the CDX model are that it is fast, cheap, and technically

Maja Čemažar, Tanja Jesenko and Urša Lampreht Tratar (eds.), *Mouse Models of Cancer: Methods and Protocols*, Methods in Molecular Biology, vol. 2773, https://doi.org/10.1007/978-1-0716-3714-2_6,
© The Author(s), under exclusive license to Springer Science+Business Media, LLC, part of Springer Nature 2024

simple, allowing for straightforward monitoring of tumor response to therapy. On the other hand, PDX tumors maintain histopathological features and genetic profiles of original patient tumors, thus providing improved clinical relevance. However, both xenograft models use immunocompromised mice, depriving the tumor of its immunological microenvironment. To overcome this limitation, humanized mouse models have been developed by engraftment of live human cells into a suitable murine host. This can be done through the transplantation of human peripheral blood mononuclear cells (PBMCs), human hematopoietic stem cells (HSCs), or specific human tissues. However, there are several pitfalls of this approach including incomplete immune reconstitution, inappropriate immune cell activity or maturation as well as donor-to-donor heterogeneity, and potential engraftment failure [1]. In contrast, the syngeneic model is established by transplanting cancer cells, either primary cells or a cell line, to an immunocompetent host mouse from the same genetic background. Therefore, syngeneic allograft models can be useful for the research of tumor–host interactions during cancer development and metastasis, functional analysis of proteins involved in tumor progression, or studies of immunotherapies, such as immune-modulators and antitumor vaccines. Disadvantages of this model include its advanced disease stage modeling and, due to its murine tumor and microenvironment, lower clinical relevance [2, 3].

In genetically modified mouse models of breast cancer, tumorigenesis occurs spontaneously in the natural microenvironment. These can be models driven by the expression of an oncogene or more complex models that mimic the genetics of human disease with spatial and temporal activation of oncogenes and/or deletion of tumor suppressor genes. In our work, we have often used the MMTV-PyMT model of breast cancer, which uses the mouse mammary tumor virus long terminal repeat promoter (MMTV-LTR) to drive the expression of polyomavirus middle T (PyMT) oncogene [4]. MMTV-LTR promoter activation is controlled by specific steroid hormones, thus restricting the oncogene expression to mammary tissue. The PyMT oncogene expression activates a signaling pathway composed of protumorigenic effectors, such as Ras, Src, and PI3K, which leads to tumor progression through distinct histological stages, which mimic human ductal breast cancer progression [5]. Neoplasms progress from benign ductal hyperplasia to a premalignant stage of ductal carcinoma in situ, followed by the transition to invasive ductal adenocarcinoma (IDC), which is marked by the breakdown of the basement membrane [5]. Gene expression profiling groups PyMT tumors with the luminal B subtype of human breast cancer [6]. The first palpable tumors appear in mice around 4 weeks of age, while all MMTV-PyMT mice aged 14 weeks exhibit large carcinomas in each of their mammary glands. MMTV-PyMT tumors also form metastases, mainly in the lungs

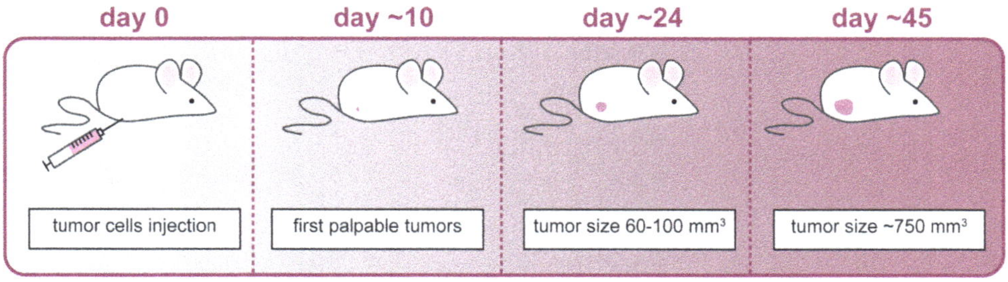

Fig. 1 Orthotopic PyMT tumor growth after tumor cells injection: first palpable tumors appear 10 days after injection. After approximately 3 weeks, tumors reach sizes 60–100 mM^3, which is appropriate for treatment. Around day 45 after injection, tumors reach sizes approx. 750 mM^3

with high incidence—at around 14 weeks of age, 100% of female mice have detectable lung metastases [4, 5, 7–9]. Another advantage of the MMTV-PyMT model is the infiltration of immune cells into the tumor, enabling the study of tumor-associated inflammation.

To study tumor response to therapy, single tumors with more control of their progression are preferred over the spontaneously formed multiple tumors in the MMTV-PyMT model. By orthotopic congenic transplantation of primary tumor cells into an immunocompetent host of the same strain, we retain the native microenvironment with an active immune response, which is required to study the pathology of the tumor microenvironment as well as the efficacy of any therapy, relying on the response of the immune cells, such as immunotherapies [10, 11]. The timeline of orthotopic tumor growth is shown in Fig. 1. Here, we provide protocols for the isolation of primary tumor cells from PyMT-MMTV cancer model and the orthotopic transplantation of these cells into congenic immunocompetent mice.

2 Materials

2.1 Isolation of Primary Tumor Cells

1. Tweezers, scissors, and scalpel (No. 10).
2. Petri dishes.
3. Enzyme cocktail: 5 mL of DNase I (0.25 mg/mL), 5 mL of Hyaluronidase Type I-S (1 mg/mL), and 5 mL of Crude Collagenase, Type IV (6 mg/mL).
4. Sterile glass beaker with glass beads and a magnetic stirring bar.
5. Magnetic plate stirrer.
6. 100 μm and 40 μm cell strainers.
7. 50 mL Falcon tubes.
8. Dulbecco's phosphate-buffered saline (DPBS).

9. Complete Dulbecco's modified Eagle medium (DMEM) (10% fetal bovine serum (FBS), 1% glutamine, and 1% penicillin/ streptomycin).
10. 15 cm cell culture dish.
11. Trypsin.
12. Trypan Blue.
13. Freezing medium: complete DMEM with 10% dimethyl sulfoxide (DMSO).
14. Cryogenic storage vials.

2.2 Orthotopic Transplantation of Primary Tumor Cells

1. Trypsin.
2. DPBS.
3. Complete DMEM.
4. DMEM.
5. 15 cm cell culture dishes.
6. 15 mL falcon tubes.
7. Trypan Blue.
8. 0.5 mL insulin syringes.
9. 70% ethanol.

3 Methods

3.1 Isolation of Primary Tumor Cells from MMTV-PyMT-Induced Mammary Carcinomas

1. Sacrifice female MMTV-PyMT transgenic mouse with a large tumor burden (i.e., 14 weeks of age) by cervical dislocation.
2. Work under aseptic conditions and using tweezers and scissors, remove the tumor mass by separating it from the skin and abdominal wall.
3. Place the tumor in a petri dish and weigh it (*see* **Note 1**), then cut the tumor into small pieces using scalpel No. 10.
4. Transfer the pieces to a sterile glass beaker with glass beads and a magnetic stirring bar. Add all of the Enzyme cocktail and incubate at 37 °C for 1 h on a magnetic hotplate stirrer with gentle stirring at approx. 100 rpm.
5. Using a pipette, transfer the suspension through a 100-µm cell strainer into a 50 mL Falcon tube.
6. Transfer the flow-through through a 40-µm cell strainer into a fresh 50 mL Falcon tube.
7. Centrifuge the flow-through at 400× g for 5 min at room temperature and discard the supernatant.

8. Add 30 mL of DPBS and gently resuspend the pellet using a pipette.
9. Centrifuge the suspension at 400× g for 5 min at room temperature and discard the supernatant.
10. Repeat **steps 8** and **9** once.
11. Resuspend the pellet in 30 mL of DMEM.
12. Divide the cell suspension into three 15 cm cell culture dishes (10 mL each).
13. Add 10 mL of DMEM to each dish.
14. Incubate the cell culture dishes in an incubator at 37 °C with 5% CO_2 overnight (*see* **Note 2**).
15. The next day remove the medium and wash the adherent cells with DPBS twice.
16. Add 3 mL of trypsin to each dish and incubate at 37 °C and 5% CO_2 for 10 min to allow cells to detach.
17. Stop the enzyme treatment with the addition of 10 mL of DMEM per dish.
18. Transfer the cell suspension to a 50 mL Falcon tube.
19. Count the cells using trypan blue staining to exclude dead cells, which stain blue.
20. Centrifuge the cell suspension at 400× g for 5 min at room temperature, discarding the supernatant.
21. Resuspend the cell suspension in a freezing medium to a concentration of 2×10^6 cells/mL.
22. Transfer the cell suspension to cryogenic storage vials, using 1 mL per vial.
23. Freeze the cells at −70 °C (*see* **Note 3**), and transfer them to liquid nitrogen storage.

3.2 Orthotopic Transplantation of Primary Tumor Cells into the Mammary Gland of Congenic Mice

1. Rapidly thaw 4×10^6 primary PyMT tumor cells (two vials of cells isolated according to Subheading 3.1) in 20 mL of DMEM and transfer them to a 15 cm cell culture dish.
2. Culture the cells at 37 °C with 5% CO_2, until they reach 70–90% confluence (i.e., 2 days).
3. Remove the medium and wash the cells with DPBS twice.
4. Perform **steps 15–18** from Subheading 3.1 to detach the cells and count them.
5. Centrifuge the cell suspension at 400× g for 5 min at room temperature, discarding the supernatant.
6. Resuspend the cells in ice-cold DMEM (without FBS) to a concentration of 1×10^6 cells/100 μL, and store them on ice.

7. Induce anesthesia in female congenic mice (FVB/N strain, i.e., 8 weeks of age), using the inhalational anesthetic isoflurane in the anesthetic chamber (*see* **Note 4**).
8. Sterilize the injection area with ethanol—i.e., the left inguinal mammary gland of the female congenic mice.
9. Gently shake the cell suspension and draw 50 μL into an insulin syringe.
10. Place the syringe with the needle on the area of the left inguinal mammary gland and enter the skin subcutaneously, positioning the needle under the nipple. Slowly inject 50 μL of the cell suspension and then slowly retract the needle.
11. Tumor diameters are measured with a digital caliper, measuring the long (a) and short diameter (b). Tumor volume is calculated using the following formula: $V = (a \times b^2) \times \pi/6$ (*see* **Note 5**).

4 Notes

1. At least 4 g of tumor tissue is needed for this protocol. With less than 4 g, split the cell suspension into two 15 cm dish plates instead of three and culture them for an additional day or two.
2. The primary PyMT tumor cells grow adherently.
3. It is recommended to use a passive freezer filled with isopropanol to ensure a slower lowering of the temperature.
4. Anesthesia induced by isoflurane inhalation persists for some minutes after removing the mice from the anesthetic chamber. In our experience, this time frame is adequate for tumor cell injection. Alternatively, anesthesia can also be induced by i.p. injection of ketamine/xylazine solution. The injection can also be done on a non-anesthetized mouse; however, it is easier to perform the procedure more precisely on an anesthetized mouse, leading to more reliable results.
5. Treatment can start approximately 3 weeks after transplantation when the tumors have reached volumes ~80–150 mM^3.

References

1. Cogels MM, Rouas R, Ghanem GE et al (2021) Humanized mice as a valuable pre-clinical model for cancer immunotherapy research. Front Oncol 11:784947
2. Holen I, Speirs V, Morrissey B et al (2017) In vivo models in breast cancer research: progress, challenges and future directions. Dis Model Mech 10:359–371
3. Sakamoto K, Schmidt JW, Wagner KU (2015) Mouse models of breast cancer. Methods Mol Biol 1267:47–71
4. Guy CT, Cardiff RD, Muller WJ (1992) Induction of mammary tumors by expression of polyomavirus middle T oncogene: a transgenic mouse model for metastatic disease. Mol Cell Biol 12:954–961

5. Lin EY, Jones JG, Li P et al (2003) Progression to malignancy in the polyoma middle T oncoprotein mouse breast cancer model provides a reliable model for human diseases. Am J Pathol 163:2113–2126
6. Pfefferle AD, Herschkowitz JI, Usary J et al (2013) Transcriptomic classification of genetically engineered mouse models of breast cancer identifies human subtype counterparts. Genome Biol 14:R125
7. Vasiljeva O, Papazoglou A, Krueger A et al (2006) Tumor cell-derived and macrophage-derived cathepsin B promotes progression and lung metastasis of mammary cancer. Cancer Res 66:5242–5250
8. Vasiljeva O, Korovin M, Gajda M et al (2008) Reduced tumour cell proliferation and delayed development of high-grade mammary carcinomas in cathepsin B-deficient mice. Oncogene 27:4191–4199
9. Vasiljeva O, Sevenich L, Reinheckel T (2021) Analyzing the role of proteases in breast cancer progression and metastasis using primary cells from transgenic oncomice. Methods Mol Biol 2294:275–293
10. Mikhaylov G, Mikac U, Magaeva AA et al (2011) Ferri-liposomes as an MRI-visible drug-delivery system for targeting tumours and their microenvironment. Nat Nanotechnol 6:594–602
11. Lerner MI, Mikhaylov G, Tsukanov AA et al (2018) Crumpled aluminum hydroxide nanostructures as a microenvironment dysregulation agent for cancer treatment. Nano Lett 18: 5401–5410

Chapter 7

Transplantable Subcutaneous Tumor Models

Simona Kranjc Brezar

Abstract

Mouse tumor models are essential in cancer research, especially in elucidating malignancy, developing prevention, diagnosis, and new therapeutic approaches. Nowadays, due to standardized ways of maintaining animal colonies and the availability of mouse strains with known genetic backgrounds and approaches to reduce the variability of tumor size between animals, transplantable mouse tumor models can be widely used in translational cancer research. Here, we describe the induction of different subcutaneous tumor models in mice, in particular xenograft and syngeneic that can be used as experimental tumor models.

Key words Subcutaneous tumor models, Mouse, Xenograft, Syngeneic, Cancer research

1 Introduction

Recently, the knowledge of cancer progression and biological characteristics of cancer cells has exceptionally increased and thus enabled the improvement of established cancer treatment as well as the development of new treatment approaches [1–3]. The *Mus musculus* is the most commonly used model to study genetic principles and human diseases over the past century, not only because of its relatively similar anatomy, physiology, and genome compared to humans, but also because of the availability, ease of handling, high reproductive rates, and relatively low cost of use [4–7]. Mouse tumor models have proven to be useful for the understanding of biological mechanisms during tumor growth and for discovering and developing improved methods of prevention, diagnosis, and cancer therapies [8–11]. For rapid screening of therapeutic approaches, most commonly are used subcutaneously transplanted syngeneic and xenografted tumors, grown in immunocompetent and immunodeficient mice, respectively [6, 11]. However, mice still have limitations in modeling human cancer, including species-specific differences, a lower degree of tumor heterogeneity compared to human tumors, and the site of tumor growth [12]. Too

Maja Čemažar, Tanja Jesenko and Urša Lampreht Tratar (eds.), *Mouse Models of Cancer: Methods and Protocols*, Methods in Molecular Biology, vol. 2773, https://doi.org/10.1007/978-1-0716-3714-2_7,
© The Author(s), under exclusive license to Springer Science+Business Media, LLC, part of Springer Nature 2024

often mice respond to experimental interventions differently than humans [6]. Thus, scientists are dealing with future challenges to generate clinically relevant mouse models that recapitulate the molecular, cellular, and genomic events of human cancers and clinical response as well as the development of technologies that allow for efficient in vivo imaging and high-throughput screening in mice [13, 14]. One possibility to meet specific tumor requirements and recapitulate proper tissue microenvironment that is known to affect tumor properties and antitumor treatment response is implanting tumors orthotopically [15–17]. However, monitoring of orthotopic tumors is more challenging and demands additional approaches that enable the tracing of tumors inside the organs, such as engineered cancer cells expressing a fluorescent protein (green, red) or firefly luciferase for tumor implantation [18–22]. Furthermore, great improvement in cancer research was achieved with the development of methods for the creation of knockout, knockin mice, and transgenic, i.e., genetically engineered mouse models, which initiated studies on early cellular and molecular events in tumor progression and metastasis and provide better preclinical models in the testing of novel therapeutic strategies in human cancer [4, 23] However, as the development of genetically engineered mouse models is very expensive, time-consuming, and challenging, research in subcutaneous tumor models is also an advantage in this respect.

A panel of tumor cell lines can be used for the generation of subcutaneous tumor models including syngeneic and xenograft [24–31]. Tumor cells are usually subcutaneously inoculated on the flank or dorsum of mice, in which the transplanted cells proliferate and form spheric structures that interact with the surrounding stroma to some extent. Subcutaneous tumors are easily accessible for treatment approaches (i.e. injection, irradiation, surgical removal,...), and the antitumor effect of tested treatments can be easily monitored by measuring them noninvasively with a caliper. In addition, subcutaneous tumors can be used for immunohistological, molecular biological, and flow cytometry analyses [29, 32, 33]. Such experimental design is cost- and time-effective. From an animal welfare point of view, it is important to limit the discomfort, pain, and distress that the tumor-bearing animals may experience during research. Thus, working with subcutaneous tumors requires more frequent on a scheduled basis observation, to assess the progress of tumor growth and/or metastasis and the general condition of the animal.

With more than two decades of experience in using animal models and excellent professional skills, our department has evaluated a variety of human (xenograft) as well as murine (syngeneic) subcutaneous tumor models that have grown in mice for research dealing with novel anticancer therapies. These tumor models were used in different approaches, i.e., increasing drug delivery, pharmacokinetics, toxicity and antitumor effectiveness of anticancer drugs, and antivascular, immunological, and radiotherapy approaches [29–41].

A list of available commonly used tumor cell lines is included in Table 1.

2 Materials

Prepare a cell suspension of tumor cells using sterile physiological saline for experimental tumor implantation into the subcutaneous tissue in the flank, back, or hind leg of the mouse (good access for therapy and tumor measurement) (Fig. 1). All procedures have to be performed according to good laboratory practice and with safety precautions. Cell lines used for tumor induction must be Mycoplasma free. Procedures on animals implement by skilled personnel.

2.1 Equipment

1. Syringe with injection needle: 0.3 mL, G29, 0.33 × 12.5 mM; 5 mL G20; 0.9 × 40 mM.
2. 50 mL and 5 mL centrifuge tube.
3. T175 Cell culture flask for adherent cells.
4. Water bath preheated at 37 °C.
5. Microscope and cell counting chamber.
6. Biological hood for sterile work.
7. Wet ice.
8. Mouse clipper.
9. Mouse cage for individually ventilated system (such as Optimice™).
10. VetFlo™ Vaporizer with induction chamber and nose cone.
11. Oxygen concentrator.
12. Weighing scale.

2.2 Reagents, Cells, and Animals

1. Tumor cell line (Table 1).
2. Cell culture media supplemented with 10% fetal bovine serum (FBS).
3. Trypsin EDTA.
4. Sterile physiological solution.
5. Sterile phosphate-buffered saline (PBS).
6. Matrigel.
7. Mouse; appropriate strain according to tumor cell line growth characteristic (Table 1).

Table 1
Subcutaneous tumor models in mice

	Solid tumor types	Cell lines	Propagation of cell line	Mouse line	N of inoculated cells
Xenograft	Human breast carcinoma	Au565 (Her2-positive)	Cell culture	NUDE (HSD: Athymic nude-Foxn1^{NU}	1×10^6
Xenograft	Human breast carcinoma	MDA-MB-231 (triple-negative)	Cell culture	NUDE (HSD: Athymic nude-Foxn1^{NU}	1×10^6
Xenograft	Human breast carcinoma	T47D (hormone receptor-positive)	Cell culture	NUDE (HSD: Athymic nude-Foxn1^{NU}	1×10^6
Xenograft	Human breast adenocarcinoma	MCF7 (estrogen receptor positive)	Cell culture	NUDE (HSD: Athymic nude-Foxn1^{NU}	1×10^6
Xenograft	Human colorectal adenocarcinoma	HT29	Cell culture	SCID-C.B-17/IcrHsdPrkdc^{scid}	5×10^5
Xenograft	Human colorectal adenocarcinoma	LoVo	Cell culture	SCID-C.B-17/IcrHsdPrkdc^{scid}	2×10^6
Xenograft	Human lung carcinoma	A549	Cell culture	SCID	1×10^7
Xenograft	Human ovarian adenocarcinoma	OVCAR5	Cell culture	NUDE	5×10^6
Xenograft	Human pharyngeal squamous cell carcinoma	FaDu (HPV negative)	Cell culture	SCID-C.B-17/IcrHsdPrkdc^{scid}	2×10^6
Xenograft	Human pharyngeal squamous cell carcinoma	2A3 (HPV positive for E6 and E7)	Cell culture	SCID-C.B-17/IcrHsdPrkdc^{scid}	5×10^6
Syngeneic	Mouse melanoma	B16F10 (highly metastatic)	Cell culture	C57Bl/6	3×10^5
Syngeneic	Mouse melanoma	B16F10-EGFP (highly metastatic)	Cell culture	C57Bl/6	3×10^5
Syngeneic	Mouse melanoma	B16F10-tomato (highly metastatic)	Cell culture	C57Bl/6	3×10^5
Syngeneic	Mouse melanoma	B16F1	Cell culture	C57Bl/6	3×10^5
Syngeneic	Mouse fibrosarcoma	SA1	Ascites	A/J	5×10^5
Syngeneic	Mouse fibrosarcoma	LPB	Cell culture	C57Bl/6	1×10^6

(continued)

**Table 1
(continued)**

	Solid tumor types	Cell lines	Propagation of cell line	Mouse line	N of inoculated cells
Syngeneic	Mouse Ehrlich-lettre ascites carcinoma	EAT	Ascites	CBA	5×10^6
Syngeneic	Mouse mammary adenocarcinoma	TS/A (highly metastatic)	Cell culture	Balb/c	2×10^6
Syngeneic	Mouse colorectal carcinoma	MC38	Cell culture	C57Bl/6	3×10^5
Syngeneic	Mouse colon carcinoma	CT26	Cell culture	Balb/c	3×10^5

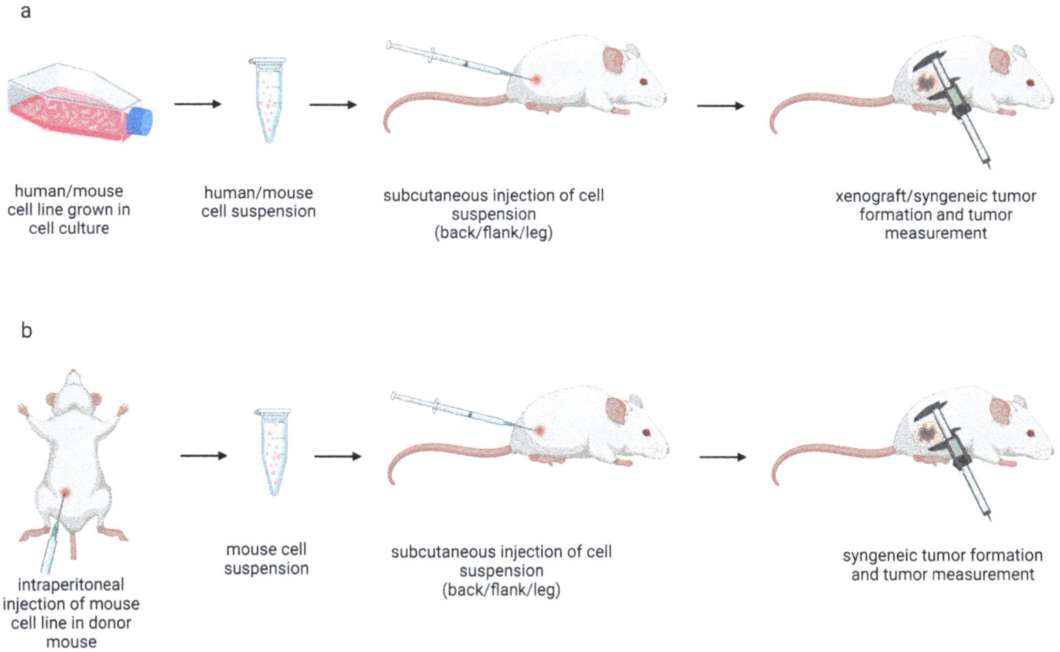

Fig. 1 Scheme of subcutaneous tumor induction and measurement. (**a**) Induction of subcutaneous tumors from cell suspension obtained in cell culture. (**b**) Induction of subcutaneous tumors from cell suspension obtained in donor animal

8. Isoflurane.
9. Skin disinfectant.

3 Methods

1. Warm the appropriate media and solutions that will be needed for culturing the cells.
2. Thaw the tumor cell line (1×10^6) at 37 °C.
3. Grow the cells to the appropriate number needed for tumor inoculation. Tumor cells can be subcultured from cell culture in cell culture flasks (*see* **Note 1**) or from the ascites in the abdominal cavity of the donor mouse (*see* **Note 2**).

   In the case of cell culture monolayer at a confluency of approximately 80%, 2 days after plating, the cells are trypsinized according to manufacturer instructions (10 mL for flask T175, 1–3 min). Following the inactivation of trypsin with an equal volume of cell culture media containing 10% of FBS, collect the cell suspension in a 50 mL centrifuge tube, and centrifuge for 5 min at 300 rpm. Wash the cell pellet with 5 mL of physiological saline and centrifuge it for 5 min at 300 rpm. Then resuspend the pellet in 2 mL of sterile physiological saline, count the cells, and prepare the appropriate cell concentration according to the tumor model (Table 1) in sterile physiological saline or in sterile physiological saline with Matrigel (*see* **Note 3**). Transfer cell suspension to a 5 mL tube and place it on wet ice till the inoculation.

   In the case of growing cells as ascites in the abdominal cavity, inject intraperitoneally 300 μL containing 10^6 cells in sterile physiological saline to the appropriate donor mouse strain (Table 1). Two days later, humanely sacrifice the donor animal, wash the abdominal cavity with 5 mL of sterile physiological saline, and collect cells by centrifugation 5 min at 1500 rpm. Resuspend the pellet in 2 mL of sterile physiological saline, count the cells, and prepare the appropriate cell concentration according to the tumor model (Table 1) in sterile physiological saline. Transfer cell suspension to a 5 mL tube and place it on wet ice till the inoculation.
4. Take the mouse from the cage and shave the area where the tumors will be inoculated (flank or back or hind leg) using a mouse clipper (*see* **Note 4**).
5. Wear protective glasses and gloves during the procedure of subcutaneous injection. The assistant holds the mouse so that it is immobilized and the injection site is exposed. Alternatively, the procedure of subcutaneous injection can be performed under anesthesia using isoflurane (*see* **Note 5**).
6. Disinfect the injection site of the skin with skin disinfectant. Slightly raise the skin fold at the injection site, insert the needle (G29) with the cut part of the tip facing up, and inject subcutaneously the tumor cell suspension: 100 μL in the flank or

back and 50 μL in the hind leg. When injected correctly, a bubble is formed under the skin (*see* **Note 6**).

7. Place the mouse back in its cage and repeat the process until all animals are injected.
8. Observe the mice twice weekly for initial tumor development and growth. In addition, monitor the animal's body weight and the general condition of the animal twice weekly (*see* **Note 7**).

4 Notes

1. Thawing of cell lines has to be quick as possible. Place the tube with frozen cell suspension into the warm water bath (37 °C). Immediately when cells are defrosted, transfer the suspension in 10 mL of preheated (37 °C) cell culture media supplemented with 10% of FBS (50 mL centrifuge tube) and centrifuge it for 5 min at 1500 rpm to remove the cell freezing media. Resuspend the pellet in 15 mL of fresh warm cell culture media supplemented with 10% of FBS and plate it on T75 cell culture flask. Culture cells for 2 days in a humidified incubator with 5% of CO_2 at 37 °C. To be sure that cells were properly defrosted and stayed viable, cells have to be cultured at least for one passage. Carefully aspirate cell culture media out of the flask, add 5–10 mL of sterile PBS into each flask to rinse off excess media. Dispense PBS down the side of the flasks to keep cells adherent. Remove PBS and add 5–10 mL of trypsin (5 mL for flask T75). Incubate at room temperature for 1–3 min. Once cells begin rounding up and can be dislodged from the flask when tapping the outside of the flask, add an equal volume of cell culture media supplemented with 10% FBS (5 mL) to inactivate the trypsin, collect the cell suspension in 50 mL conical tube, and centrifuge it for 5 min at 1500 rpm. Carefully aspirate the media, resuspend the cell pellet in 2 mL of fresh cell culture media, and count the cells. Then plate cells appropriate number of cells on culture flask T175 containing 20 mL of cell culture media supplemented with 10% FBS. If cells remain attached, the flasks can be incubated at 37 °C with careful monitoring of cell lifting. Avoid overtrypsinizing cells. Cells used for the tumor induction have to be mycoplasma free. To obtain subcutaneous tumors with properly developed tumor vasculature, low concentration of cells should be injected so that the tumor initiation process with the formation of tumor vessels is slow.
2. Thawing of cell lines has to be quick as possible. Place the tube with frozen cell suspension into the warm water bath (37 °C). Immediately when cells are defrosted, transfer the suspension

in 10 mL of preheated (37 °C) cell culture media supplemented with 10% of FBS (50 mL centrifuge tube) and centrifuge it for 5 min at 1500 rpm to remove the cell freezing media. Resuspend the pellet in 300 μL of fresh warm physiological saline (10^6 cells) and inject intraperitoneally into the donor mouse, where cells grow in the abdominal cavity for 2 days. Animal well-being should be inspected every day; however, according to our experience 2 days after inoculation, animals did not develop any serious clinical signs.

3. Growing xenografts could be more delicate. Precisely, some cells have to be prepared in a sterile physiological saline containing 50% of Matrigel, i.e., OVCAR5, MCF7. Matrigel contains a mixture of major basement-membrane extracellular matrix proteins (e.g., laminin, collagen IV, entactin, and the heparan sulfate proteoglycan perlecan), growth factors, and many enzymes that help cells to grow subcutaneously at the beginning of tumor formation. Note that all needed material has to be cooled down at −20 °C (tubes, needles, syringes); after thawing the Matrigel, it has to be kept on wet ice and mixed with cell suspension just prior beginning of injections.
4. Animals should be shaved the day before subcutaneous injection so that the mice are not irritated when inoculating the cell suspension.
5. To reduce their risk of puncture with cells, mice are anesthetized when using human tumor cell lines (potentially infectious, possible transplantation [42, 43] or performing the procedure alone with isoflurane in an induction chamber with the isoflurane level at 2–3% until unconsciousness is achieved and then lowered to 1.5–2%. When animals are unconscious, pull them out one at a time and place them on a nose cone. Clean the injection site at the skin with skin disinfectant, slightly raise the skin fold at the injection site, insert the needle (G29) with the cut part of the tip facing up, and inject subcutaneously the tumor cell suspension: 100 μL in the flank or back and 50 μL in the hind leg.
6. Before each withdrawal of cells into the syringe, mix the cells well. Inject slowly and wait for additional 5 s to maintain the bubble (tumor placement). Injection must be subcutaneous if intradermal; otherwise, skin necrosis will develop during tumor growth.
7. Depending on the tumor cell line, tumors may take 1–8 weeks to appear. Animals with tumors of 6 mm in maximum diameter have to be evaluated and the tumor size measured and recorded daily until removal from the study. Furthermore, the humane endpoints must be determined in advance. Animals with tumors reaching 12 mm in maximum diameter or those with

ulcerated tumors, impaired mobility, ≥20% body weight loss, ataxia, hunched posture, or labored breathing have to be removed from the study and humanely euthanized [9].

References

1. Hanahan D (2022) Hallmarks of cancer: new dimensions. Cancer Discov 12:31–46
2. Pearlman AH, Hwang MS, Konig MF et al (2021) Targeting public neoantigens for cancer immunotherapy. Nat Cancer 2:487–497
3. Faubert B, Solmonson A, DeBerardinis RJ (2020) Metabolic reprogramming and cancer progression. Science 368:eaaw5473
4. Walrath JC, Hawes JJ, Van Dyke T, Reilly KM (2010) Genetically engineered mouse models in cancer research. In: Advances in cancer research, vol 106. Academic Press, pp 113–164
5. Waterston RH, Lindblad-Toh K, Birney E et al (2002) Initial sequencing and comparative analysis of the mouse genome. Nature 420: 520–562
6. Perlman RL (2016) Mouse models of human disease: an evolutionary perspective. Evol Med Public Health 2016:170–176
7. Rosenthal N, Brown S (2007) The mouse ascending: perspectives for human-disease models. Nat Cell Biol 9:993–999
8. Cheon DJ, Orsulic S (2011) Mouse models of cancer. Annu Rev Pathol 6:95–119
9. Workman P, Aboagye EO, Balkwill F et al (2010) Guidelines for the welfare and use of animals in cancer research. Br J Cancer 102: 1555–1577
10. Ireson CR, Alavijeh MS, Palmer AM et al (2019) The role of mouse tumour models in the discovery and development of anticancer drugs. Br J Cancer 121:101–108
11. Kelland LR (2004) Of mice and men: values and liabilities of the athymic nude mouse model in anticancer drug development. Eur J Cancer 40:827–836
12. Tammela T, Sage J (2020) Investigating tumor heterogeneity in mouse models. Annu Rev Cancer Biol 4:99–119
13. Wade CM, Daly MJ (2005) Genetic variation in laboratory mice. Nat Genet 37:1175–1180
14. Lee JS, Chu IS, Mikaelyan A et al (2004) Application of comparative functional genomics to identify best-fit mouse models to study human cancer. Nat Gene 36:1306–1311
15. Hoffman RM (1999) Orthotopic metastatic mouse models for anticancer drug discovery and evaluation: a bridge to the clinic. Investig New Drugs 17:343–360
16. Killion JJ, Radinsky R, Fidler IJ (1998) Orthotopic models are necessary to predict therapy of transplantable tumors in mice. Cancer Metastasis Rev 17:279–284
17. Francia G, Cruz-Munoz W, Man S et al (2011) Mouse models of advanced spontaneous metastasis for experimental therapeutics. Nat Rev Cancer 11:135–141
18. Klerk CPW, Overmeer RM, Niers TMH et al (2007) Validity of bioluminescence measurements for noninvasive in vivo imaging of tumor load in small animals. Biotechniques 43: S7–S13, S30
19. Madero-Visbal RA, Colon JF, Hernandez IC et al (2012) Bioluminescence imaging correlates with tumor progression in an orthotopic mouse model of lung cancer. Surg Oncol 21: 23–29
20. Hoffman RM (2008) A better fluorescent protein for whole-body imaging. Trends Biotechnol 26:1–4
21. Hoffman RM (2005) The multiple uses of fluorescent proteins to visualize cancer in vivo. Nat Rev Cancer 5:796–806
22. Huang L, Bommireddy R, Munoz LE et al (2021) Expression of tdTomato and luciferase in a murine lung cancer alters the growth and immune microenvironment of the tumor. PLoS One 16:e0254125
23. Lampreht Tratar U, Horvat S, Cemazar M (2018) Transgenic mouse models in cancer research. Front Oncol 8:268
24. Jung J (2014) Human tumor xenograft models for preclinical assessment of anticancer drug development. Toxicol Res 30:1–5
25. Olson B, Li Y, Lin Y et al (2018) Mouse models for cancer immunotherapy research. Cancer Discov 8:1358–1365
26. Negro G, Aschenbrenner B, Kranjc Brezar S et al (2020) Molecular heterogeneity in breast carcinoma cells with increased invasive capacities. Radiol Oncol 54:103–118
27. Berne S, Čemažar M, Frangež R et al (2018) APS8 delays tumor growth in mice by inducing apoptosis of lung adenocarcinoma cells expressing high number of α7 nicotinic receptors. Mar Drugs 16:367
28. Kranjc Brezar S, Mrak V, Bosnjak M et al (2020) Intratumoral gene electrotransfer of

plasmid DNA encoding shRNA against melanoma cell adhesion molecule radiosensitizes tumors by antivascular effects and activation of an immune response. Vaccine 8:135
29. Kranjc Brezar S, Prevc A, Niksic Zakelj M et al (2020) Synergistic effect of cisplatin chemotherapy combined with fractionated radiotherapy regimen in HPV-positive and HPV-negative experimental pharyngeal squamous cell carcinoma. Sci Rep 10:1563
30. Bozic T, Sersa G, Kranjc Brezar S et al (2021) Gene electrotransfer of proinflammatory chemokines CCL5 and CCL17 as a novel approach of modifying cytokine expression profile in the tumor microenvironment. Bioelectrochemistry 140:107795
31. Sedlar A, Kranjc S, Dolinsek T et al (2013) Radiosensitizing effect of intratumoral interleukin-12 gene electrotransfer in murine sarcoma. BMC Cancer 13:38
32. Prosen L, Hudoklin S, Cemazar M et al (2016) Magnetic field contributes to the cellular uptake for effective therapy with magnetofection using plasmid DNA encoding against Mcam in B16F10 melanoma in vivo. Nanomedicine 11:627–641
33. Dolinsek T, Sersa G, Prosen L et al (2015) Electrotransfer of plasmid DNA encoding an anti-mouse endoglin (CD105) shRNA to B16 melanoma tumors with low and high metastatic potential results in pronounced antitumor effects. Cancers (Basel) 8:3
34. Remic T, Sersa G, Levpuscek K et al (2022) Tumor cell-based vaccine contributes to local tumor irradiation by eliciting a tumor model-dependent systemic immune response. Front Immunol 13:974912
35. Vidic S, Markelc B, Sersa G et al (2010) MicroRNAs targeting mutant K-ras by electrotransfer inhibit human colorectal adenocarcinoma cell growth in vitro and in vivo. Cancer Gene Ther 17:409–419
36. Hudej R, Miklavcic D, Cemazar M et al (2014) Modulation of activity of known cytotoxic ruthenium(III) compound (KP418) with hampered transmembrane transport in electrochemotherapy in vitro and in vivo. J Membr Biol 247:1239–1251
37. Prevc A, Kranjc S, Cemazar M et al (2018) Dose-modifying factor of radiation therapy with concurrent cisplatin treatment in HPV-positive squamous cell carcinoma: a preclinical study. Radiat Res 189:644–651
38. Sersa G, Jarm T, Kotnik T et al (2008) Vascular disrupting action of electroporation and electrochemotherapy with bleomycin in murine sarcoma. Br J Cancer 98:388–398
39. Kranjc S, Tevz G, Kamensek U et al (2009) Radiosensitizing effect of electrochemotherapy in a fractionated radiation regimen in radiosensitive murine sarcoma and radioresistant adenocarcinoma tumor model. Radiat Res 172: 677–685
40. Kranjc S, Cemazar M, Grosel A et al (2005) Radiosensitising effect of electrochemotherapy with bleomycin in LPB sarcoma cells and tumors in mice. BMC Cancer 5:115–281
41. Serša G, Kranjc S, Čemažar M (2000) Improvement of combined modality therapy with cisplatin and radiation using electroporation of tumors. Int J Radiat Oncol Biol Phys 46:1037–1041
42. Gugel EA, Sanders ME (1986) Needle-stick transmission of human colonic adenocarcinoma. N Engl J Med 315(23):1487–1986
43. Geraghty RJ, Capes-Davis A, Davis JM et al (2014) Guidelines for the use of cell lines in biomedical research. Br J Cancer 111:1021–1046

Chapter 8

Preclinical Mouse Metastatic Model Established Through Induced Lung Metastases

Katja Uršič Valentinuzzi, Gregor Serša, and Urška Kamenšek

Abstract

Metastatic disease is the major cause of cancer death, and the lung is one of the most common sites of cancer metastases. To investigate systemic antitumor effects or protective potential of local therapies, mouse models with induced metastases are indispensable in preclinical cancer research. Here, we describe the protocol for the metastatic mouse model established through induced 4T1 mammary carcinoma metastases. With minor prior optimization, it can be applied to other tumor cell lines of interest.

Key words Metastases, Lungs, Mouse models, Cancer, Lung colonization assay

1 Introduction

More than 90% of cancer-related mortality is due to disease progression through metastases [1–3]. In contrast, preclinical evaluation of new cancer treatments often examines only regression of the primary tumor. Primary tumors and metastases tend to respond differently to therapies, making it difficult to predict outcomes in patients with advanced metastatic disease [4]. Therefore, predictive, standardized, and well-defined models of systemic disease are crucial to facilitate translational research. Such models not only aid in preclinical drug development but also enable the study of systemic immune-mediated antitumor responses.

Rodents, especially mice, are the gold standard in cancer research. Many murine tumor models metastasize spontaneously. Spontaneous murine metastases models recapitulate all steps of the metastatic cascade and have proven to be extremely valuable in understanding the biology of metastases. However, due to shortcomings such as the long interval to metastatic onset and interanimal variables, these models are not very useful for preclinical testing of potential therapies, where induced metastases models come into play [5]. Several sites can be used for vascular injection of tumor

Maja Čemažar, Tanja Jesenko and Urša Lampreht Tratar (eds.), *Mouse Models of Cancer: Methods and Protocols*, Methods in Molecular Biology, vol. 2773, https://doi.org/10.1007/978-1-0716-3714-2_8,
© The Author(s), under exclusive license to Springer Science+Business Media, LLC, part of Springer Nature 2024

cells in mice, which then define the site of metastases. These include intravenous induction of lung metastases, intracardiac induction of brain and bone metastases, intrasplenic induction of metastases in lymph nodes and liver metastases, intratibial induction of bone metastases as well as intraperitoneal induction of mesentery metastases [6]. Compared with spontaneous metastases models, induced metastases models bypass the initial steps of the metastatic cascade and only model the late stages of metastatic disease. However, the systemic antitumor effects of local therapies and the link between immune cells and metastases can be efficiently studied [7].

Here, we describe our protocol for the induction of mouse syngeneic lung metastases, which can be used to investigate systemic antitumor effects or the protective potential of local therapies (Fig. 1). Lung metastases are induced by tail vain injection of tumor cells. Then, the treatment under study (i.e., local treatment with systemic effect or systemic treatment) is applied. When the systemic efficacy of a local therapy is studied, primary tumors can be induced in parallel with the induction of metastases. After a predetermined period of time, the lungs are harvested and fixed, and metastases are macroscopically counted. The comparison of the metastatic burden between the control group and the treated group provides information about the antimetastatic efficacy of the tested therapy. In addition, the harvested lungs can be histologically sectioned and specifically stained to allow microscopic assessment. Alternatively, noninvasive imaging techniques such as ultrasound, microcomputed tomography, small-animal positron emission tomography (PET), small-animal computed tomography (CT), single-photon emission computed tomography (SPECT), as well as fluorescence and bioluminescence imaging can be used for longitudinal monitoring of metastases [8, 9]. The last two techniques prerequisite the use of genetically modified cell lines expressing reporter genes that can drastically affect the immunogenicity of the model, so they should be used with special caution [10–12].

The protocol described refers to 4T1 mammary carcinoma, a transplantable tumor model syngeneic to Balb/c mice, which is also known to metastasize spontaneously from the induced tumors to multiple distant sites, including lymph nodes, blood, liver, lung, brain, and bone. Compared to spontaneous metastases, intravenously induced lung metastases represent a more reproducible and time-efficient model. This model also reduces the number of animals and the need for constant monitoring of metastatic spread, which requires the use of the aforementioned imaging techniques. In addition to 4T1, we and others have successfully used similar protocols for the induction of LPB, SA1 [13], and B16F10 metastases [14, 15]. Therefore, the protocol described here can be readily adopted for other tumor cell lines of interest with minor prior optimization.

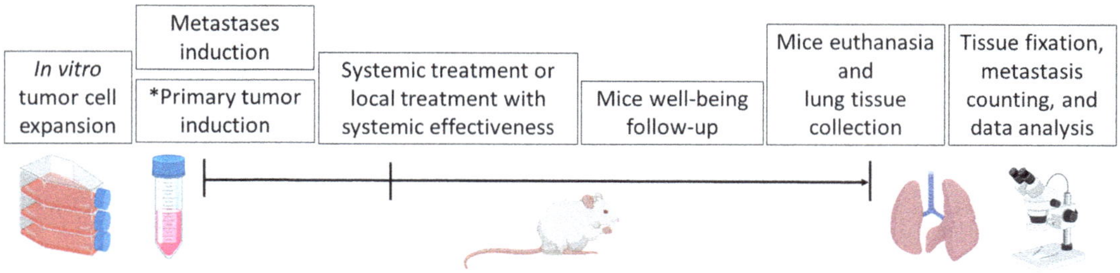

Fig. 1 Schematic presentation of the protocol for the preclinical mouse metastatic model established through induced lung metastases. *When the systemic efficacy of a local therapy is studied, primary tumors can be induced in parallel with the induction of metastases

2 Materials

2.1 Cell Suspension

1. Mouse mammary carcinoma 4T1 cells.
2. Culturing medium: advanced Roswell Park Memorial Institute (RPMI) 1640 medium containing 5% fetal bovine serum (FBS), 10 mM L-glutamine (Glutamax), 100 U/mL penicillin, and 50 mg/mL gentamicin.
3. Buffers: sterile 0.25% trypsin-EDTA solution pH 7.2 (for 1000 mL: 900 mL Hank's balanced salt solution, 100 mL 2.5% trypsin, 5.4 mL 7.5% $NaHCO_3$, 0.2 g EDTA), sterile phosphate-buffered saline pH 7.2 (1 × PBS; for 1000 mL: 8 g NaCl, 0.2 g KCl, 1.15 g Na_2HPO_4, 0.2 g KH_2PO_4, and up to 1000 mL distilled water), physiological solution (0.9% NaCl).
4. Consumables: culturing flasks (T-75, T-182), serological pipettes (5 mL, 10 mL, 25 mL, 50 mL), pipette tips (0.1–1000 μL), centrifuge tubes (15 mL, 50 mL), microcentrifuge tubes (1.5 mL, 2 mL), disinfectant.
5. Equipment: laminar flow hood, centrifuge, pipettes, pipetboy, inverted microscope, protective clothing, and gloves.

2.2 Injection of Tumor Cells

1. Ice in a small container for short-term storage of cell suspension.
2. Balb/c mice.
3. 70% ethanol, disinfectant.
4. Consumables: syringe (G27; 0.4 × 13), pipette tips, gauze.
5. Equipment: induction restrainers, shaving machine, pipettes, protective clothing and gloves, sharps container, heat lamp.

2.3 Histopathological Examination of Metastases

1. Buffers: Bouin's fixative (75 mL saturated aqueous solution of picric acid, 25 mL of 40% aqueous solution of formaldehyde and 5 mL glacial acetic acid) and physiological solution (0.9% NaCl).
2. Consumables: sample containers.
3. Equipment: stereomicroscope, tweezers, petri dish, protective clothing, and gloves.

3 Methods

3.1 Cell Suspension

Before you start, ensure that the cells are authenticated and mycoplasma free (*see* **Note 1**).

1. Warm-up the culturing medium and trypsin-EDTA solution to 37 °C before use.
2. Culture 4T1 cells in complete medium under standard culture conditions: in a humidified chamber at 37 °C, 5% CO_2. Expand the cells in T-75 (10 mL media; up to 5×10^6 cells) or T-182 (15 mL media; up to 15×10^6) culture flasks to 70–80% confluency. Determine confluency using an inverted microscope.
3. Remove the culturing medium and wash the cells once with 1× PBS (T-75: 5 mL; T-182: 10 mL).
4. Add trypsin-EDTA to the flasks (T-75: 3 mL; T-182; 5 mL) to thoroughly cover all cells and incubate at 37 °C for up to 1 min or until cells have detached.
5. Immediately after, add the complete culturing medium with FBS to inactivate the trypsin-EDTA. Use the same volume as trypsin-EDTA.
6. Transfer the single-cell suspension from the flask to a centrifuge tube using a 25 mL sterile pipette.
7. Pellet the cells by centrifugation 300 × *g*, 5 min, and room temperature.
8. Discard the supernatant and resuspend the cells in up to 5 mL of physiological solution. The volume varies depending on the cell number.
9. Count the cells using a hemocytometer or an automated cell counter.
10. Prepare a cell suspension containing 3×10^6 cells/ml in physiological solution.
11. Keep the cell suspension on ice until injection.

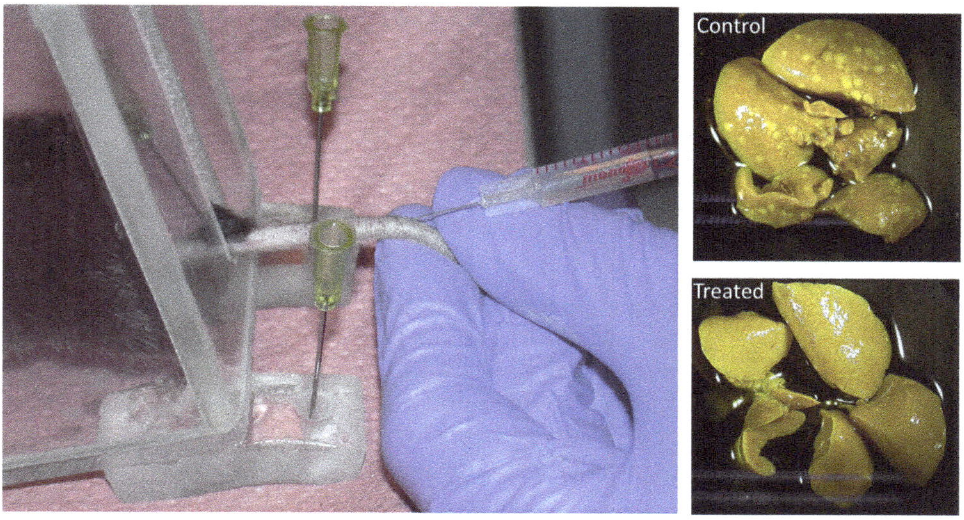

Fig. 2 Preclinical mouse metastatic model established through induced lung metastases. Left: mouse in induction restrainer with tail exposed. Right: fixed lungs of untreated (control) and treated mice

3.2 Induction of Metastases

All procedures, including experiments with mice, should comply with national laws, regulations, or official guidelines on animal experimentation, as well as directives. Plan the experiments following the 3Rs principle (*see* **Note 2**).

1. Place a mouse in an induction restrainer and properly secure the mouse with the tail exposed (Fig. 2).
2. For successful injection, the tail veins should be visible and dilated. If not, use a heating lamp or hot water for dilatation (*see* **Note 3**).
3. Disinfect the tail with 70% ethanol.
4. Mix the cell suspension well and load a syringe. Degas a syringe and inject 0.1 mL of the cell suspension into one of the lateral tail veins of Balb/c mice (*see* **Note 4**). Cells (3×10^5) are sufficient to induce 4T1 metastases in all injected mice (*see* **Note 5**).
5. Optional: Induce primary tumors following your standard protocol (*see* **Note 6**).

3.3 Histopathological Examination of Metastases

1. Follow the well-being of the mice until the onset of metastases (*see* Note 7).
2. Humanely euthanize the mouse (*see* **Note 8**).
3. Harvest the lungs (*see* **Note 9**).
4. After dissection, rinse the lungs in a Petri dish with physiological solution, dry them with a clean paper towel, and place them in a container with Bouin's solution (3–5 mL).
5. Incubate in Bouin's solution overnight.

6. Transfer the lungs to 70% ethanol.
7. Count the metastases on the lung surface under a stereomicroscope.
8. Microscopic evaluation (*see* **Note 10**).

4 Notes

1. Contaminated and misidentified cell lines can compromise the reproducibility and reliability of experiments and lead to incorrect scientific conclusions. Therefore, a growing number of scientific journals and funding agencies require the implementation and reporting of both. We recommend the use of cell cultures from renowned cell banks, implementing consistent (certificated) quality control. This generally includes testing for authenticity as well as for mycoplasma contamination. Further handling of the cells could lead to misidentification of the cells and mycoplasma contamination. Therefore, regular authenticity and contamination testing is essential. There are many commercially available tests that can be performed in any better equipped cell laboratory [16, 17]. The International Cell Line Authentication Committee (ICLAC) provides guidelines for best practice. Otherwise, cell banks also offer both services.
2. Animals are still indispensable in translational research. Because of ethical issues, ethics committees should approve animal experimentation prior to initiation. Countries regulate animal experimentation differently; therefore, animal experimentation should comply with national laws, regulations, or official guidelines. The common denominator of animal experimentation is the 3Rs principle (replacement, reduction, and refinement) [18]. To ensure consistent and detailed performance of experiments involving live animals, the PREPARE guidelines (Planning Research and Experimental Procedures on Animals: Recommendations for Excellence) and the ARRIVE guidelines (Animal Research: Reporting of In Vivo Experiments) cover a checklist of information to ensure transparent and thorough planning and reporting [19]. All animal experiments were performed in accordance with the guidelines for animal experiments of the EU directives, the ARRIVE guidelines, and the approval of the Ministry of Agriculture, Forestry and Food of the Republic of Slovenia (permits no. U34401–1/2015/43 and U34401–3/2022/11).
3. Specialized equipment is essential for proper immobilization. There are several commercially available restrainers (Fig. 3). The procedure can also be performed under isoflurane

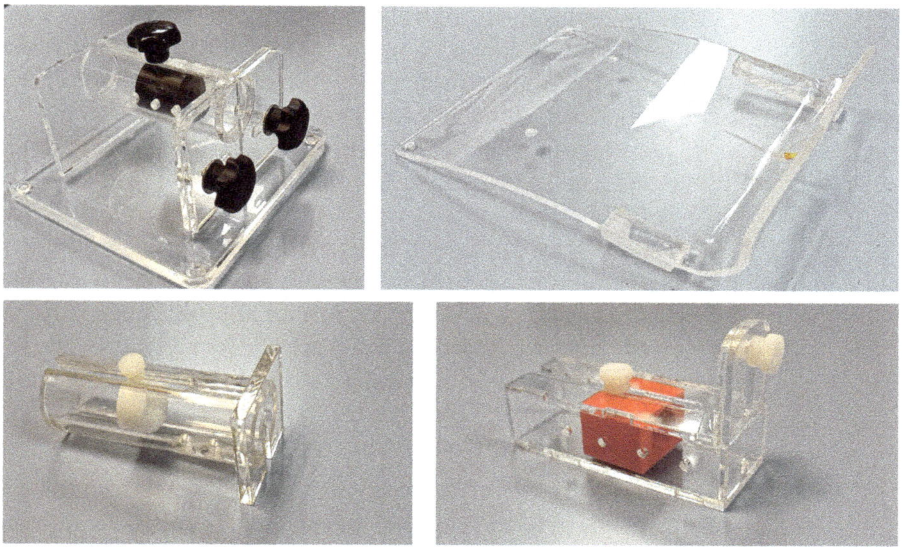

Fig. 3 Available induction restrainers

inhalation anesthesia; however, no refinement regarding pain and distress has been demonstrated [20].

Restraints are used to restrict the movement of the animal while leaving the tail freely accessible. Different sizes of restraints enable their use on mice of different ages and sizes. Especially with small animals, it can be difficult to prevent the mouse from turning around. Therefore, we found paper towels useful to provide additional restraint for the animal.

To achieve vasodilation that allows injection into the tail vein, the procedure is often combined with heat treatment. Specifically, we investigated two different procedures: immersion of the tail in warm water or local infrared exposure. The latter proved to be easier, faster and more effective. However, special care should be taken to localize the heating to minimize the stress caused by (over) heating the animal.

4. Tail vein injection requires adequate practical skills before it can be used safely and routinely. It is classified as a mild procedure and is routinely performed without animal anesthesia. However, be prepared for the mouse to react and move during the procedure.

   Before placing the animal in a restrainer, prepare all the equipment needed. Place the animal in the restrainer, hold the warmed tail with your nondominant hand, rotate it gently and locate one of the two lateral tail veins. Use 70% ethanol to clean the skin and increase the visibility of the veins. Start with the injection in the middle third of the tail and move cranially if the injection was not successful in the first attempt. Place the needle with the bevel facing up and slide the needle a few millimeters through the skin and into the tail vein. Ensure that that the needle is completely parallel to the vein and do not go too deep into the tail. Do not pull back the plunger prior to injection when injecting cell suspensions as it may result in clumping of the cells. Instead, start by injecting a very small volume of cell suspension to test whether you are in the vein. Low injection pressure (no resistance while injecting) and blanching of the vein indicate that needle is in the vein. Unsuccessful injection will result with a subcutaneous swelling. After the injection, apply pressure with a sterile gauze at the injection site until the bleeding has stopped. After the procedure, discard the used needle into a sharps container, move the animal to its home cage and observe animal for few minutes. Complications after the properly executed procedure are rare.

5. The onset of macroscopically visible metastases can be adjusted by varying the number of injected tumor cells. Furthermore, the protocol described here can be readily adopted for other tumor cell lines of interest with minor prior optimization.
6. Consider this optional step when evaluating the systemic effect of local therapies. The exact time interval between the induction of the metastases and the primary tumors should be preliminary determined for each model, considering the time that tumors take to grow and whether you want to study protection against metastasis formation or the effect on already established metastases.
7. In the 4T1 model, the time of mouse euthanasia and lung collection was between 14 and 17 days. This was based on preliminary experiments evaluating different time points from 7 days on.
8. Carbon dioxide is the most commonly used agent for rodent euthanasia. However, a number of studies have examined the histological effects of CO_2 on the lung. Terminal CO_2 inhalation has been shown to cause alveolar extravasation (hemorrhage into the tissue), pulmonary edema, hemorrhage, pulmonary edema, and emphysema [21]. Therefore, our method of choice for euthanasia in this protocol would be cervical dislocation. The effectiveness of dislocation can be verified by palpation of the cervical tissue: a separation between the occipital condyles and the first cervical vertebra should be clearly palpable.
9. Use needles to secure mouse to the dissecting board and position it in a dorsal recumbency with full extension of pelvic and pectoral limbs. Apply 70% ethanol to mouse fur to avoid hair contamination during the dissection. Start with the incision of the skin and abdomen at the ventral midline and continue cranially and caudally to expose peritoneal cavity and the

xiphoid process. Use scissors to open the rib cage and expose the entire thoracic cavity. Thereafter, use scissors to cut the trachea and tweezers to dissect the lungs.

10. Quantification of lung metastases can also be performed via microscopic evaluation with prior paraffin embedding, sectioning, and hematoxylin and eosin (H&E) staining of the lung tissue.

Acknowledgments

The research was supported by the Slovenian Research Agency (grant numbers P3-0003 and Z3-2651).

References

1. Jamil A, Kasi A (2022) Lung metastasis. StatPearls, Treasure Island
2. Massagué J, Obenauf AC (2016) Metastatic colonization. Nature 529:298. https://doi.org/10.1038/NATURE17038
3. Dillekås H, Rogers MS, Straume O (2019) Are 90% of deaths from cancer caused by metastases? Cancer Med 8:5574. https://doi.org/10.1002/CAM4.2474
4. Merlino DJ, Johnson JM, Tuluc M et al (2020) Discordant responses between primary head and neck tumors and nodal metastases treated with neoadjuvant nivolumab: correlation of radiographic and pathologic treatment effect. Front Oncol 10:1. https://doi.org/10.3389/FONC.2020.566315/FULL
5. Francia G, Cruz-Munoz W, Man S et al (2011) Mouse models of advanced spontaneous metastasis for experimental therapeutics. Nat Rev Cancer 11:135. https://doi.org/10.1038/NRC3001
6. Gómezgómez-Cuadrado L, Tracey N, Ma R et al (2017) Mouse models of metastasis: progress and prospects. https://doi.org/10.1242/dmm.030403
7. Janssen LME, Ramsay EE, Logsdon CD, Overwijk WW (2017) The immune system in cancer metastasis: friend or foe? J Immunother Cancer 5:79. https://doi.org/10.1186/s40425-017-0283-9
8. Lee HN, Kim S, Park S et al (2022) Quantification and visualization of metastatic lung tumors in mice. Toxicol Res 38:503–510. https://doi.org/10.1007/s43188-022-00134-4
9. Marien E, Hillen A, Vanderhoydonc F et al (2017) Longitudinal microcomputed tomography-derived biomarkers for lung metastasis detection in a syngeneic mouse model: added value to bioluminescence imaging. Lab Investig 97:24–33. https://doi.org/10.1038/LABINVEST.2016.114
10. Bresser K, Dijkgraaf FE, Pritchard CEJ et al (2020) A mouse model that is immunologically tolerant to reporter and modifier proteins. Commun Biol 3(1):273. https://doi.org/10.1038/s42003-020-0979-0
11. Serganova I, Blasberg RG (2019) Molecular imaging with reporter genes: has its promise been delivered? J Nucl Med 60:1665–1681. https://doi.org/10.2967/jnumed.118.220004
12. Baklaushev VP, Kilpeläinen A, Petkov S et al (2017) Luciferase expression allows bioluminescence imaging but imposes limitations on the orthotopic mouse (4T1) model of breast cancer. Sci Rep 7(1):7715. https://doi.org/10.1038/s41598-017-07851-z
13. Tevz G, Kranjc S, Cemazar M et al (2009) Controlled systemic release of interleukin-12 after gene electrotransfer to muscle for cancer gene therapy alone or in combination with ionizing radiation in murine sarcomas. J Gene Med 11:1125–1137. https://doi.org/10.1002/jgm.1403
14. Sf Guimarães F, Andrade LF, Martins ST et al (2010) *In vitro* and *in vivo* anticancer properties of a Calcarea carbonica derivative complex (M8) treatment in a murine melanoma model. BMC Cancer 10:113. https://doi.org/10.1186/1471-2407-10-113
15. Gautam A, Waldrep JC, Densmore CL et al (2002) Growth inhibition of established B16-F10 lung metastases by sequential aerosol delivery of p53 gene and 9-nitrocamptothecin.

Gene Ther 9:353–357. https://doi.org/10.1038/sj/gt/3301662

16. Corral-Vázquez C, Aguilar-Quesada R, Catalina P et al (2017) Cell lines authentication and mycoplasma detection as minimun quality control of cell lines in biobanking. Cell Tissue Bank 18:271. https://doi.org/10.1007/S10561-017-9617-6
17. Marx V (2014) Cell-line authentication demystified. Nat Methods 11(5):483–488. https://doi.org/10.1038/nmeth.2932
18. Lee KH, Lee DW, Kang BC (2020) The 'R' principles in laboratory animal experiments. Lab Anim Res 36(1):45. https://doi.org/10.1186/S42826-020-00078-6
19. Percie Du Sert N, Hurst V, Ahluwalia A et al (2020) The ARRIVE guidelines 2.0: updated guidelines for reporting animal research. BMC Vet Res 16:1–7. https://doi.org/10.1186/S12917-020-02451-Y/TABLES/2
20. Resch M, Neels T, Tichy A et al (2019) Impact assessment of tail-vein injection in mice using a modified anaesthesia induction chamber versus a common restrainer without anaesthesia. Lab Anim 53(2):190–201. https://doi.org/10.1177/0023677218786982
21. Conlee KM, Stephens ML, Rowan AN et al (2005) Carbon dioxide for euthanasia: concerns regarding pain and distress, with special reference to mice and rats. Lab Anim 39(2):137–161. https://doi.org/10.1258/0023677053739747

Chapter 9

In Vivo Wound Healing Model for Characterization of Gene Electrotransfer Effects in Mouse Skin

Špela Kos, Tanja Jesenko, and Tanja Blagus

Abstract

Wound healing is a complex biological response to injury characterized by a sequence of interdependent and overlapping physiological actions. To study wound healing and cutaneous regeneration processes, the complexity of wound healing requires the use of animal models. In this chapter, we describe the protocol to generate skin wounds in a mouse model. In the mouse splinted excisional wound model, two full-thickness wounds are firstly created on the mouse dorsum, which is followed by application of silicone splint around wounded area. A splinting ring tightly adheres to the skin around full-thickness wound, preventing wound contraction and replicating human processes of re-epithelialization and new tissue formation. The wound is easily accessible for treatment as well as for daily monitoring and quantifying the wound closure.

This technique represents valuable approach for the study of wound healing mechanisms and for evaluation of new therapeutic modalities. In this protocol, we describe how to utilize the model to study the effect of gene electrotransfer of plasmid DNA coding for antiangiogenic molecules. Additionally, we also present how to precisely regulate electrical parameters and modify electrode composition to reach optimal therapeutic effectiveness of gene electrotransfer into skin around wounded area.

Key words Skin, Full-thickness wound, Splint, Mouse model, Gene electrotransfer, Plasmid DNA, Antiangiogenic molecules

1 Introduction

Dermal wound healing is a complex physiological response proceeding with multistep phases; beginning with hemostasis and inflammation followed by cellular proliferation, extracellular matrix formation, angiogenesis and tissue remodeling, and ultimately scar formation [1–3]. To study wound healing and cutaneous regeneration processes, the complexity of wound healing necessitates the use of animal models. The laboratory mouse remains by far the most commonly used animal model for wound healing research. Nevertheless, important factor to consider when designing mouse experiments are significant differences between mouse and human skin and differential processes involved in wound regeneration

Maja Čemažar, Tanja Jesenko and Urša Lampreht Tratar (eds.), *Mouse Models of Cancer: Methods and Protocols*, Methods in Molecular Biology, vol. 2773, https://doi.org/10.1007/978-1-0716-3714-2_9,
© The Author(s), under exclusive license to Springer Science+Business Media, LLC, part of Springer Nature 2024

[4]. In particularly, mouse skin is unique in having a *Panniculus carnosus* layer, i.e., a subcutaneous muscle layer, which produces rapid wound contractions following injury. In contrast to mouse skin, where contraction accounts for a large part of wound closure, human wounds heal via re-epithelialization and granulation tissue formation [4–6].

To overcome the differential healing process in mouse and humans, we have utilized *a splinted excisional wound model*. Briefly, in this model, two full-thickness excisional wounds extending through the subcutaneous tissue on the dorsum on each side of the midline are created. A silicone splint is tightly attached to the skin around the wound, preventing local skin contractions [7, 8]. The wound therefore heals through re-epithelialization and new tissue formation, approximating a process occurring in humans. Following intradermal or topical treatment, a transparent occlusive dressing is applied. By removing the dressing, the wound bed can be easily accessed to apply further treatment or daily monitoring and imaging of the wounds.

The complex biologic process of wound repair becomes abnormal in numerous diseases. This cost-effective and easy to perform model can be utilized to assessed wound healing in context of several pathophysiologies, such as diabetes mellitus and arterial or venous insufficiency. In this protocol, we represent the excisional splinted model for studying the effects of intradermal injection of plasmid DNA encoding antiangiogenic molecule followed by electroporation, a method called gene electrotransfer. Gene electrotransfer is a safe and efficient nonviral gene delivery method based on application of controlled electric pulses applied to cells or tissues [9]. Gene therapy techniques delivering exogenous angiogenic factors and cytokines to skin are currently being investigated to increase wound perfusion and healing [10]. To take full advantage of electroporation mediated delivery of therapeutic molecules to skin, it is important to establish an efficient and safe delivery system. Thus, the described model provided us a tool for investigating optimal electric conditions for skin gene electrotransfer by monitoring the effects of gene electroporation and antiangiogenic plasmids delivery on wound closure [11, 12].

2 Materials

2.1 Experimental Animals

1. BALB/c female mice (6–8 weeks old) from a commercial breeder (*see* **Note 1**).

2.2 Splints

1. Outline 15 mm circles on 0.5 mm thick silicone sheeting. Use scissors, circle cutters, or biopsy punch to create silicone discs.

2. Center a 6 mm biopsy punch in the middle of 15 mm circle to create a "donut-shaped" disc, which will be used as a splint.
3. Autoclave splints prior to the surgery.
4. Apply instant bonding adhesive (e.g., Loctite Super Attak Glue) to fix the splint to the skin.

2.3 Surgical Materials and Equipment

1. Hair removal (depilatory) cream.
2. Electric clipper for hair removal.
3. Sterile gauze and cotton swabs (*see* **Note 2**).
4. 70% ethanol.
5. Saline solution (0.9% NaCl).
6. Povidone–iodine solution.
7. 5 mm biopsy punch.
8. Tissue scissors and forceps (surgical grades).
9. 29-G insulin grade syringe for anesthetic and plasmid injection.
10. Heating pad.
11. 5-0 Mersilk nonabsorbable sutures.
12. Transparent occlusive dressing.

2.4 Electroporation Devices

1. Electroporator (e.g., Cliniporator (IGEA, s.r.l., Carpi, Italy)).
2. Noninvasive multielectrode array (MEA) consisting of six spring-loaded pins arranged in circular mesh and spaced 3.5 mm apart (Iskra Medical, Podnart, Slovenia). Electrode is described in **Note 3**.

2.5 Reagents

1. Plasmid DNA: 80 μL of 2 mg/mL plasmid DNA per wound (*see* **Note 4**).
2. 0.3 mg/kg analgesic Butorphanol.
3. General anesthetic: mixture of 1 mg/mL Ketamine, 5 mg/mL Xylazin, and 0.4 mg/mL Acepromazine dissolved in saline solution for injections.
4. MiliQ water.
5. Eye drops for moisturizing mouse eyes during the procedure.

2.6 Monitoring of the Wound Healing Process

1. 2% Isoflurane and small animal anesthesia system.
2. Stereomicroscope for image acquisition.
3. Computer software for quantification of wound area.
4. ImageJ software or similar for image processing.

3 Methods

Before surgical procedure, prepare all the necessary material and clean working surfaces with disinfectant.

3.1 Anesthesia and Operative Preparation

1. Weigh an experimental mouse and induce general anesthesia by intraperitoneal injection of prepared anesthetic. The volume of injected anesthetic depends on mouse weight. Approximate volumes for BALB/c mice are calculated as follows: 17.5 g ~ 65 μL; 18.5 g ~ 70 μL; 19.5–20.5 g ~ 75 μL; 21–22 g ~ 80–90 μL.
2. Ensure the deep pedal reflexes of the mouse are suppressed and place the mouse in the prone position.
3. Prepare the operative region by removing hair from dorsal side of the mice with an electric clipper.
4. Apply depilatory cream for no longer than 2 min. Wet gauze swabs can be used to remove all cream and remaining fur.
5. Wipe the skin with 10% povidone–iodine. After drying, place the mouse on a heating pad covered with sterile cotton gauze (Fig. 1a).
6. Apply eye drops for moisturizing mouse eyes during the procedure.

3.2 Excision of Wounds

1. Make two full-thickness wounds extending through the subcutaneous tissue on the dorsum on each side of the midline using a 5 mm biopsy punch (*see* **Note 5**). Briefly, lift the skin from the dorsal line (Fig. 1b), push the sterile biopsy punch into the skin (Fig. 1c) with a twisting motion left and right to excise two circle pieces of the skin at both sides instantaneously (Figs. 1d and 2a).
2. Clean the wounds with sterile cotton swabs.

3.3 Treatment

1. Inject 80 μL of plasmid DNA intradermally on four sites around each wound (4 × 20 μL) using 29-G insulin grade syringe (Fig. 2b). Inject the same volume of MiliQ water or control plasmid DNA around the wound in mice included in the control group (*see* **Note 6**).
2. Immediately after plasmid injection, place the MEA covering the wound (Fig. 2c, d) and apply electric pulses by electroporator. The optimal selection of electrical parameters is described in **Note 7**.
3. Repeat the treatment on the other wound.

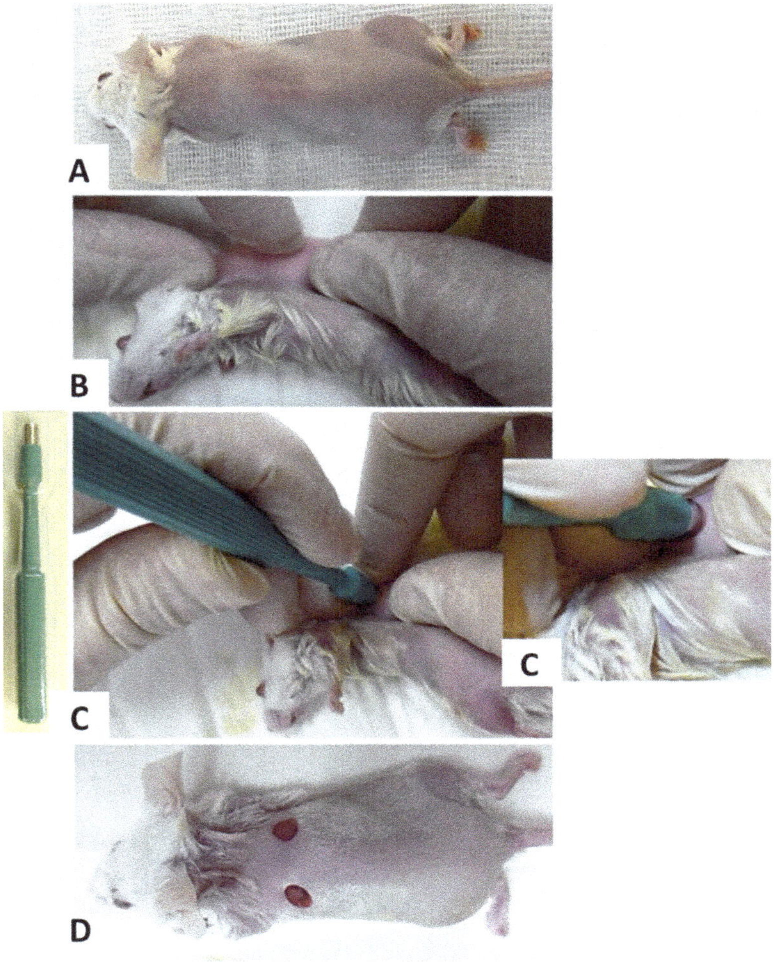

Fig. 1 Excision of wounds. Place the mouse on heating pad covered with sterile cotton gauze (**a**). Lift the skin from the dorsal line (**b**), push the sterile biopsy punch into the skin (**c**) and excise two circle pieces of the skin on the dorsum on both side of the midline (**d**)

3.4 Splinting of Wounds

1. Rinse the splint with 70% ethanol (Fig. 3a).
2. After drying (Fig. 3b), apply instant bonding adhesive to one side of silicone splint (Fig. 3c).
3. Center the splint over the wound (Fig. 3d) and anchor the splint with interrupted 5-0 Mersilk nonabsorbable sutures (Fig. 3e, f).
4. Repeat the splinting process on the other wound.
5. Rinse the wounds with saline solution.
6. Cover the wound with a transparent occlusive dressing (e.g., Tegaderm) (Fig. 4).

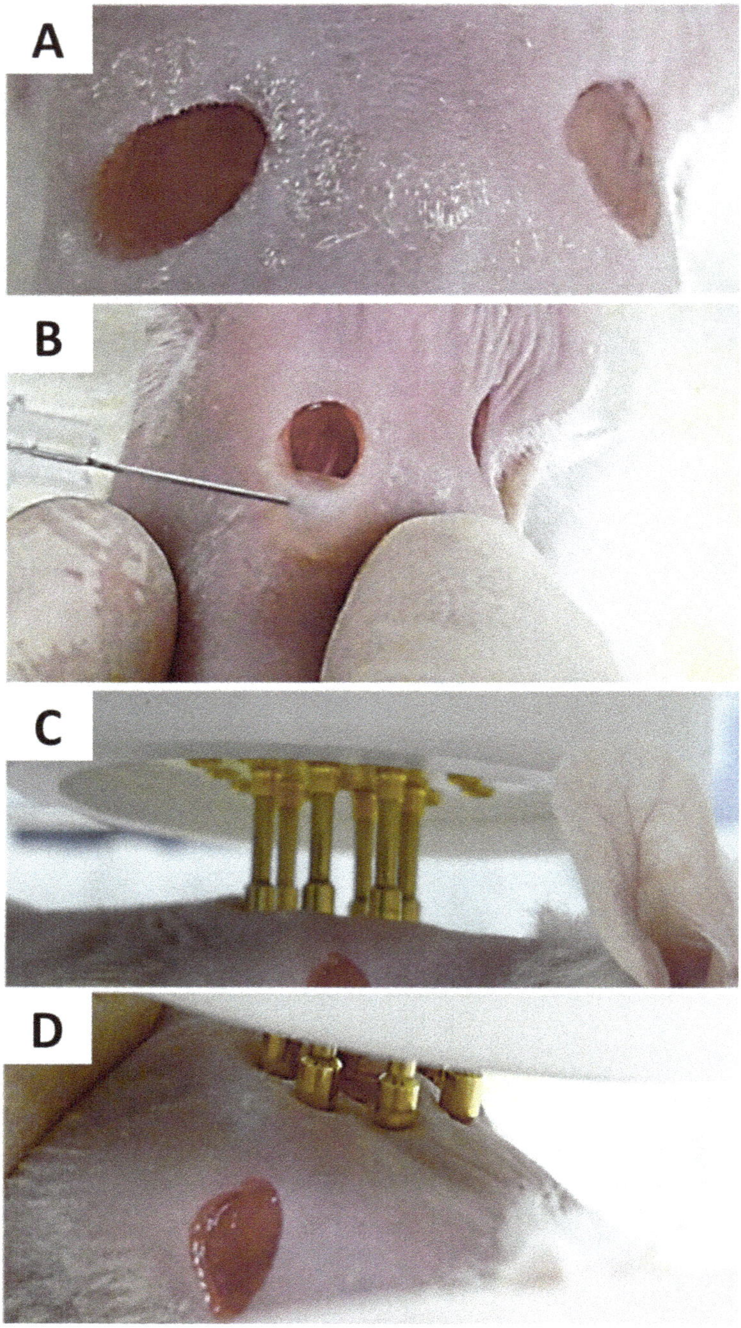

Fig. 2 Treatment—gene electrotransfer. Inject plasmid DNA intradermally in four sites around each wound (**a** and **b**). Immediately after plasmid injection, catch each wound in between MEA electrodes (**c** and **d**) and apply electric pulses

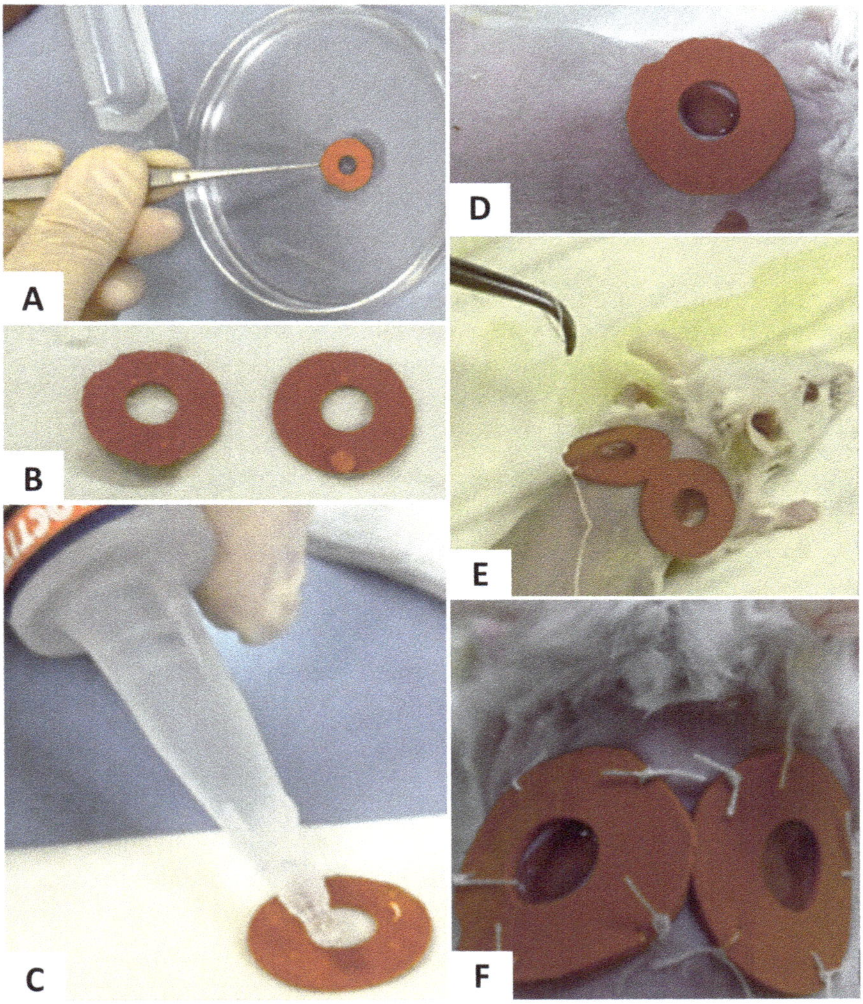

Fig. 3 Splinting of wound. Rinse the splint with 70% ethanol (**a**). After drying (**b**), apply immediate bonding adhesive to one side of silicone splint (**c**). Center the splint over the wound (**d**) and anchor the splint with sutures (**e** and **f**). Repeat the splinting process on the other wound

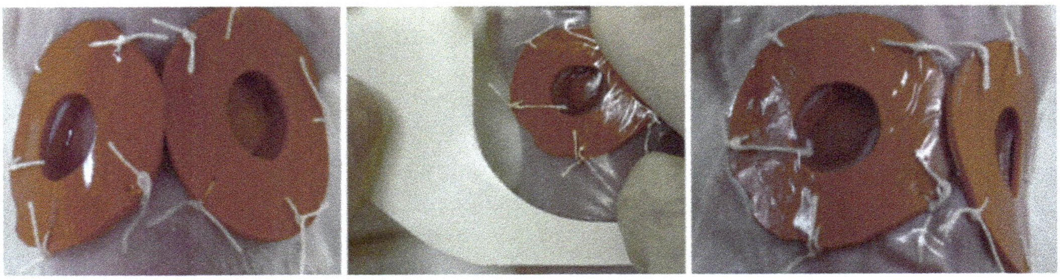

Fig. 4 Covering the wound with a transparent occlusive dressing

3.5 Postoperative Management

1. After the surgery, inject 50 μL of Butorphanol (0.3 mg/kg) intramuscularly to reduce postoperative pain. Repeat the injection of Butorphanol after 24 h.
2. Cage mice individually. Maintain them on heating pads until fully recovered (*see* **Note 8**).
3. Monitor animals twice daily for manifestations of pain and weight loss. In our experiments, no gross behavioral displays of pain or weight loss were observed.

3.6 Monitoring of the Wound Healing Process

Immediately after the splinting, capture an image of the wounds using stereomicroscope equipped with digital camera (image taken at day 0). Subsequently, record the wounds every other day until full closure of the wounds (*see* **Note 9**).

1. Induce general anesthesia of mice with 2% isoflurane using small animal anesthesia system.
2. Put the mouse under the stereomicroscope and gently peel back the transparent dressing with forceps.
3. Capture the image of the wound at both sides.
4. Reapply a clean transparent dressing and monitor the mouse until fully recovered.

3.7 Analysis of the Results

1. Quantify wound area using appropriate software (e.g., AxioVision software (Carl Zeiss Microscopy, LLC, NY, USA)).
2. Express the results as the percentage of wound coverage compared with day 0 postsurgery and normalize them to the control group treated with MiliQ water or control plasmid DNA.

4 Notes

1. In the experiments, 6- to 8-week-old mice were included. Usage of younger mice ensures that the skin surface is intact.
2. To achieve maximal sterile conditions for the experimental procedure, autoclave gauze and cotton swabs prior to the surgery.
3. For the delivery of plasmid DNA into skin, pulses were applied using non-invasive multi-electrode array (MEA), consisting of 6 spring-loaded pins arranged in the circle with the distance of 3.5 mm between each other. Two electric pulses between each electrode pair in frequency of 5 kHz were delivered during the treatment. The electrodes were provided by Iskra Medical (Podnart, Slovenia). With MEA, the applied voltage was minimized by maintaining a short electrode distance. This diminished or eliminated muscle twitching and pain associated with the application of the pulsed electric field [13].

4. Up to date, several different protein-coding genes important for skin wound healing have been identified. In our study, different plasmids coding for therapeutic molecules with anti-angiogenic actions were used: plasmids encoded shRNA against endoglin (CD105), shRNA against MCAM, plasmid encoded IL-12 [12], and peptide LL-37 [11, 14]. Other plasmids could be used accordingly.
5. Create the wounds on either side of mouse's midline at the level of the front legs, preventing the mouse to bit and remove the splint.
6. To avoid cross-contamination or systemic effects of plasmid DNA, both wounds on the left and right flank received same treatment.
7. The amplitude and duration of electric pulses used for gene electrotransfer are two critical parameters, which can affect the efficiency of transgene expression as well as tissue damage. We tested two different types of electric pulses; short HV pulses with an amplitude-over-distance ratio of 1600 V/cm and duration 100 μs, and long LV pulses with amplitude-over-distance ratio of 170 V/cm and duration 150 ms. It was demonstrated that electrotransfer parameters could regulate the depth of transfection in the skin and could essential contribute to the duration of gene expression as well as regulate the local or systemic distribution of the transcribed protein. Thus, it is of the utmost importance to select the optimal electrical parameters according to the mode of action of the transcribed molecule. We demonstrated that for plasmids encoding molecules with a local mode of action, such as shRNA against endoglin or shRNA against MCAM, the best effectiveness was obtained with HV pulses, which transfect the cells in the superficial mouse skin layers. In that way, the HV pulses would restrict the distribution of molecules with a local mode of action locally in the skin, thus avoiding possible systemic side effects due to their distribution in the bloodstream. In contrast, with molecules that have paracrine and systemic modes of action, such as IL-12, we obtained better effectiveness with LV pulses that promote the transfection of deeper skin layers [12].
8. After the surgery, cage mice individually and provide them food soaked in water until they are fully recovered.
9. At the completion of the experiments, wound closure, morphological architecture, and degree of neovascularization can be assessed by immunohistochemistry and gene expression analysis. The protocols are described elsewhere [6].

Acknowledgments

The authors acknowledge financial support from the state budget of the Slovenian Research Agency (Program no. P3-0003).

References

1. Chereddy KK, Coco R, Memvanga PB et al (2013) Combined effect of PLGA and curcumin on wound healing activity. J Control Release 171:208–215. https://doi.org/10.1016/j.jconrel.2013.07.015
2. Chereddy KK, Lopes A, Koussoroplis S et al (2015) Combined effects of PLGA and vascular endothelial growth factor promote the healing of non-diabetic and diabetic wounds. Nanomedicine 11:1975–1984. https://doi.org/10.1016/J.NANO.2015.07.006
3. Braiman-Wiksman L, Solomonik I, Spira R, Tennenbaum T (2007) Novel insights into wound healing sequence of events. Toxicol Pathol 35:767–779. https://doi.org/10.1080/01926230701584189
4. Gurtner GC, Wong VW, Sorkin M et al (2011) Surgical approaches to create murine models of human wound healing. J Biomed Biotechnol 2011:1. https://doi.org/10.1155/2011/969618
5. Wu J, Landén NX (2020) Investigation of skin wound healing using a mouse model. Methods Mol Biol 2154:239–247. https://doi.org/10.1007/978-1-0716-0648-3_20
6. Dunn L, Prosser HCG, Tan JTM et al (2013) Murine model of wound healing. J Vis Exp 2013:1–6. https://doi.org/10.3791/50265
7. Wang X, Ge J, Tredget EE, Wu Y (2013) The mouse excisional wound splinting model, including applications for stem cell transplantation. Nat Protoc 8:302–309. https://doi.org/10.1038/nprot.2013.002
8. Galiano RD, Michaels VJ, Dobryansky M et al (2004) Quantitative and reproducible murine model of excisional wound healing. Wound Repair Regen 12:485–492. https://doi.org/10.1111/J.1067-1927.2004.12404.X
9. Yarmush ML, Golberg A, Sersa G et al (2014) Electroporation-based technologies for medicine: principles, applications, and challenges. Annu Rev Biomed Eng 16:295–320. https://doi.org/10.1146/annurev-bioeng-071813-104622
10. Ferraro B, Cruz YL, Coppola D, Heller R (2009) Intradermal delivery of plasmid VEGF (165) by electroporation promotes wound healing. Mol Ther 17:651–657. https://doi.org/10.1038/Mt.2009.12
11. Kos S, Vanvarenberg K, Dolinsek T et al (2017) Gene electrotransfer into skin using noninvasive multi-electrode array for vaccination and wound healing. Bioelectrochemistry 114:33–41. https://doi.org/10.1016/j.bioelechem.2016.12.002
12. Kos S, Blagus T, Cemazar M et al (2016) Electrotransfer parameters as a tool for controlled and targeted gene expression in skin. Mol Ther Nucleic Acids 5:e356. https://doi.org/10.1038/mtna.2016.65
13. Kos S, Blagus T, Cemazar M et al (2015) Utilization of multi-array electrodes for delivery of drugs and genes in the mouse skin. IFMBE Proc 53:321–324
14. Steinstraesser L, Lam MC, Jacobsen F et al (2014) Skin electroporation of a plasmid encoding hCAP-18/LL-37 host defense peptide promotes wound healing. Mol Ther 22:734–742. https://doi.org/10.1038/mt.2013.258

Chapter 10

Partial-Volume Irradiation of Murine Tumors

Ziva Modic, Bostjan Markelc, and Tanja Jesenko

Abstract

Radiotherapy is a widely used approach for cancer treatment. However, delivering a single high dose of radiation to bulky tumors can be challenging due to the toxicities induced in the surrounding healthy tissue. To overcome this issue, a nonuniform high dose can be delivered using partial-volume tumor irradiation or spatially fractionated radiotherapy (SFRT). Moreover, SFRT has the potential to induce a stronger antitumor immune response compared to traditional radiotherapy due to the preservation of immune cells in the unirradiated tumor regions. There are several SFRT approaches, including GRID therapy, three-dimensional GRID therapy (LATTICE), microbeam radiation therapy (MRT), and **S**tereotactic **B**ody **R**adiation **T**herapy for **PA**rtial **T**umor irradiation targeting exclusively the **HY**poxic segment (SBRT-PATHY). The following protocol describes partial-volume tumor irradiation, a technique that enables dose delivery to only a part of the tumor in mice using an X-ray generator and collimators of different dimensions that limit the size of the irradiation field.

Key words Radiotherapy, Partial-volume irradiation, Spatially fractionated radiotherapy, Mouse model, Bulky tumor

1 Introduction

Radiotherapy is one of the standard approaches for treatment of several cancer types. In addition to its direct cell-killing effect, which is achieved through DNA damage and the induction of mitotic cell death, radiation can also induce immunogenic cell death and lead to several immunologically important changes [1, 2]. However, delivering a high, homogenous dose of irradiation in a single fraction is challenging especially in bulky tumors, due to the toxicities it can induce in the surrounding healthy tissue. Additionally, since lymphocytes are more sensitive to radiation [3] with less than 40% viable CD4 T helper cells and CD8 T cells after 2 Gy whole-body irradiation in C57Bl/6 mice [4], spatially fractionated radiotherapy (SFRT) could potentially induce stronger antitumor immune response compared to the irradiation of the entire tumor

Maja Čemažar, Tanja Jesenko and Urša Lampreht Tratar (eds.), *Mouse Models of Cancer: Methods and Protocols*, Methods in Molecular Biology, vol. 2773, https://doi.org/10.1007/978-1-0716-3714-2_10,
© The Author(s), under exclusive license to Springer Science+Business Media, LLC, part of Springer Nature 2024

volume, due to the sparing of immune cells in the unirradiated or low-dose tumor areas.

Therefore, different approaches of partial-volume tumor irradiation or SFRT have been developed, where the dose is nonuniformly distributed resulting in peak and valley dose areas [5]. One of the first developed SFRT approaches is GRID therapy, which delivers the dose through open fields of a perforated Cerrobend or brass screen known as GRID block or GRID collimator, resulting in a honeycomb pattern of dose delivery. GRID blocks are either custom-made or commercially available with different ratios of open to close areas, different hole diameters, and different center-to-center hole spacings [6]. An equivalent dose distribution as with GRID block can be achieved by using a multileaf collimator, which is easily modifiable, but the time needed to deliver the same dose is longer [7]. For treatment of bulky deep-seated tumors, three-dimensional GRID therapy (LATTICE) has been developed, where the tumor is irradiated with multiple irradiation beams resulting in several high-dose spheres within the tumor volume [8]. Stereotactic body radiation therapy (SBRT) has been combined with SFRT in SBRT-PATHY which targets only the hypoxic fraction of the tumor [9, 10].

Another approach of SFRT, which has been tested in preclinical animal models to date, is microbeam radiation therapy (MRT), in which the irradiation beam is divided into several coplanar high-energy beams with the width in the range between 20 and 100 μm. Even though the results in small preclinical animal models are promising [11], there are still some technical obstacles to successful translation of the approach into clinical use, such as patient-positioning systems that must provide the necessary spatial precision for the desired dose distribution [12].

Partial-volume tumor irradiation has also been used as a form of SFRT in mouse and rat models [13, 14]. Partial-volume tumor irradiation in immunocompetent mice induced comparable tumor responses both in 67NR breast cancer model and Lewis lung carcinoma model, which Markovsky et al. [13] attributed to immune response activation.

The protocol describes a technique of partial-volume tumor irradiation on in vivo mouse models, by using an X-ray generator and a custom-made set up consisting of a lead table that protects the mouse from the irradiation, and a collimator that enables the delivery of the irradiation dose to a small, defined square irradiation field.

2 Materials

2.1 Tumor Models and Cell Culture

1. Tumor cells and appropriate cell culture medium (*see* **Note 1**).
2. 1× Phosphate-buffered saline (PBS).
3. 0.25% Trypsin solution.
4. Normal saline (0.90% w/v NaCl).
5. Neubauer counting chamber or automated cell counter.
6. Experimental animals (*see* **Note 2**).
7. Syringes and 27-gauge needles for tumor induction.
8. Digital caliper and digital scale to assess tumor volumes and animal weight.

2.2 Anesthesia

1. Inhalation anesthesia device with induction chamber and anesthesia cone mask (*see* **Note 3**).
2. Isoflurane.
3. Waste anesthesia gas canisters.
4. Heating pad connected to a compatible temperature controller.
5. Eye drops.

2.3 Irradiation Device

1. In our experiments, we used Gulmay 225 X-ray system with 0.55 mm Cu and 1.8 mm Al filtering and 0.97 Gy/min dose rate.
2. Lead table with a hole for inserting the tube with a collimator (Fig. 1a, b).
3. Tubes with collimators of various dimensions (Fig. 1c).

3 Methods

3.1 Heterotopic Tumor Induction

1. Harvest the cells when they reach 70–80% confluency. Wash the cells with 1× PBS and trypsinize them with 0.25% trypsin at 37 °C. When all the cells detach, inactivate the trypsin by adding double the amount of complete cell culture medium. To pellet the cells, centrifuge at 300 × *g*, 5 min.
2. Wash the cells with normal saline, centrifuge at 300 × *g*, 5 min.
3. Resuspend the cells in normal saline, count using a Neubauer chamber or automated cell counter. Resuspend at a suitable concentration and keep on ice.
4. Inject 100 μL of the cell suspension subcutaneously into the shaved flank region of 8- to 12-week-old C57Bl/6 mice (*see* **Notes 4** and **5**).

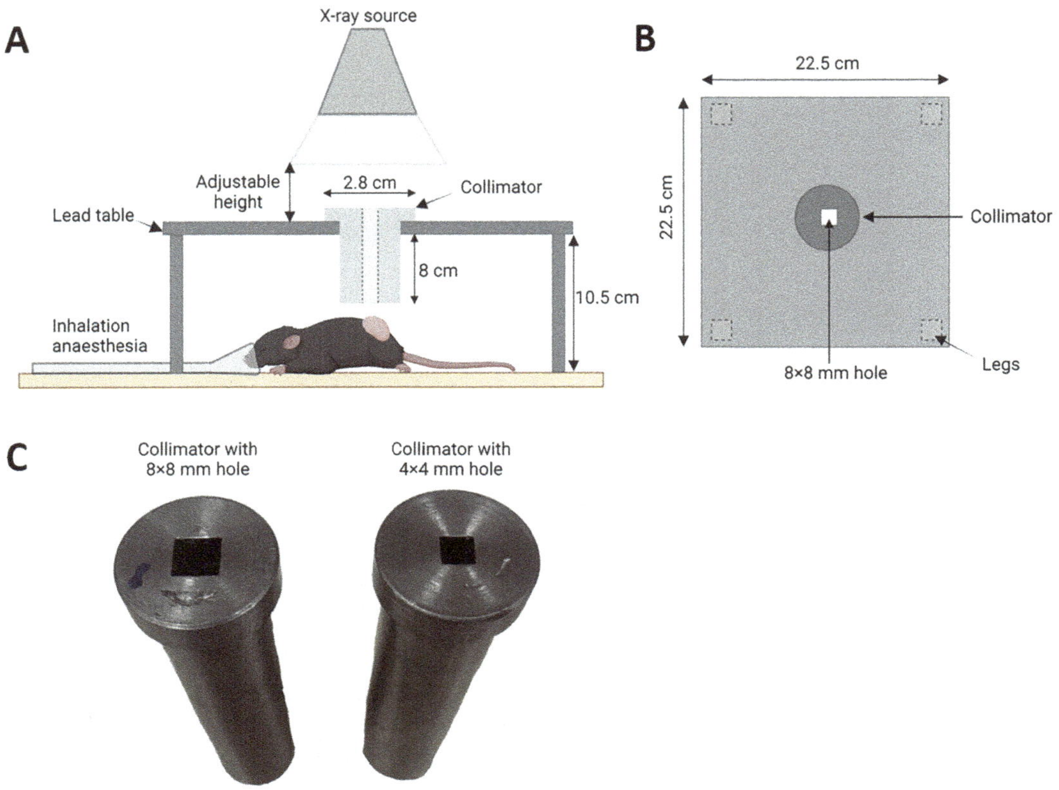

Fig. 1 Partial-volume irradiation set-up. (**a**) Side view of the partial-volume irradiation set-up. Irradiation to the desired tumor area is delivered through the collimator, inserted into the hole in the lead table, that protects the animal from irradiation. (**b**) Top view of the lead table with inserted collimator. (**c**) Examples of two collimators with different hole dimensions

5. Wait until the tumors reach the desired volume. In our experiments, formula for ellipsoid is used for tumor volume calculation ($V = a \times b \times c \times \pi/6$, where a, b, and c are perpendicular diameters of the tumor).

3.2 Preparation of the Irradiation Device and Anesthesia

1. Warm-up the irradiation device according to the device manual.
2. Prepare the anesthesia device according to the device manual (in case of SommoSuite® Low-Flow Anesthesia System, fill the glass syringe with isoflurane solution and connect it to the device, warm-up the vaporizer, and connect the induction chamber and anesthesia cone mask).
3. Prepare and prewarm the heating pad to 37 °C.

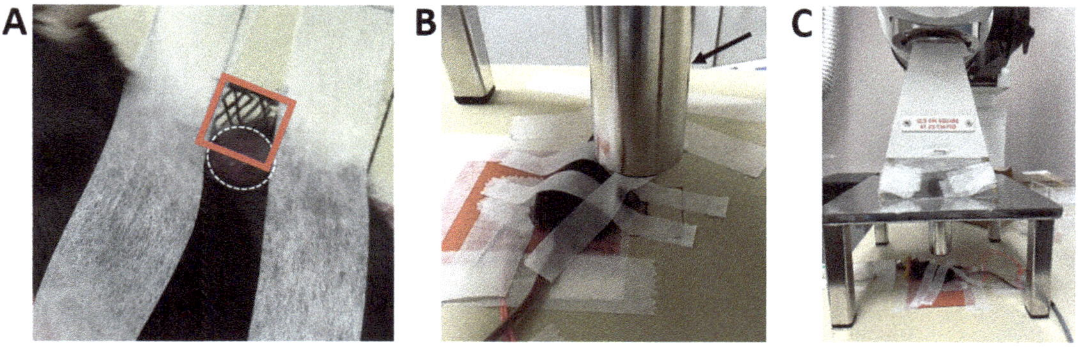

Fig. 2 Mouse fixation for partial tumor volume irradiation. (**a**) Using a micropore tape, the mouse should be fixed so that only one part of the tumor (denoted with the white dotted line) is exposed to the irradiation field (denoted with the red rectangle). (**b**) The collimator above the tumor (marked with the black arrow) enables the delivery of the irradiation dose to a specific area. (**c**) Before delivering the desired irradiation dose to the tumor, the X-ray tube should be lowered to align with the lead shielding table

3.3 Partial-Volume Tumor Irradiation

1. Anesthetize the mouse in the anesthesia induction chamber.
2. When anesthetized, transfer the mouse to the heating pad and fit the mouse muzzle to the anesthesia cone mask (*see* **Note 6**). Apply eye drops to the eyes to prevent corneal drying.
3. Using the micropore tape, position the mouse so that only one part of the tumor will be exposed to the irradiation field (Fig. 2a) (*see* **Note 7**).
4. Place the lead shielding table with the inserted collimator above the mouse (Fig. 2b). If necessary, rotate the collimator to precisely target just the desired part of the tumor (*see* **Note 8**).
5. Lower the X-ray tube to align with the lead shielding table (Fig. 2c).
6. Deliver the desired irradiation dose (*see* **Note 9**).
7. Allow the animal to recover from anesthesia before transferring it to the cage with other animals.
8. Monitor the mice daily and measure tumor volume three times per week to determine the tumor growth kinetics. Additional assays can be performed to determine the effect of partial-volume tumor irradiation depending on the scope of the research and laboratory infrastructure (e.g., *see* **Notes 10** and **11**).

4 Notes

1. In our experiments, we used the murine oral squamous cell carcinoma cell line MOC2, which is syngeneic to C57Bl/6NCrl mice. MOC2 cell culturing medium consists of Iscove's Modified Dulbecco's Medium (IMDM)/Ham's F12 Nutrient

Mixture, in a ratio of 2:1, supplemented with 5% (v/v) fetal bovine serum (FBS), 100 U/ml penicillin, 100 μg/ml streptomycin, 5 μg/ml insulin, 40 ng/ml hydrocortisone, and 5 ng/ml epidermal growth factor (EGF).

2. The mouse strain should genetically match the tumor cell line used for tumor induction. In our experiments, we used C57Bl/6NCrl mice.
3. In our experiments, we used the SommoSuite® Low-Flow Anesthesia System (Kent Scientific, CT, USA).
4. If using MOC2 cells, prepare cell suspension with 3×10^6 cells/ml. This way, each mouse is injected with 3×10^5 MOC2 cells for tumor induction.
5. Shave the mice the day before tumor induction to reduce the stress posed on the animals. Hold the mouse firmly in one hand and use electric hair trimmer to shave the flank region.
6. Isoflurane dose for anesthesia maintenance is around 1.5–2% and should be adjusted for each mouse based on observation of the animal—e.g., in case of rapid breathing increase the isoflurane dose, in case of gasping reduce the isoflurane dose.
7. The size of the irradiation field is dependent on the dimensions of the collimator and should be chosen based on the volume of the tumor being irradiated. In our experiments, we used mice with tumor volumes between 50 and 60 mm^3 and an 8×8 mm collimator to target approximately half of the tumor.
8. Proper positioning of the tumor can be verified by applying a light-source through the collimator and making sure the desired part of the tumor is illuminated. If you notice the tumor has moved out of the irradiation field, use more micropore tape to fix the tumor securely.
9. Using the set-up described and 200 kV and 9.2 A, the dose rate is 0.97 ± 0.03 Gy/min. The dose distribution is presented in Fig. 3a, b.
10. To visualize the induced DNA damage (such as double-strand breaks) in the irradiated part of the tumor, sacrifice the mouse 1 h after irradiation and prepare the tumor for immunofluorescent labeling with an anti-γH2AX antibody.
11. To determine changes in immune cell populations, use flow cytometric analysis of control and irradiated tumors. Sacrifice the animals at time points when you expect changes in immune cell populations (e.g., 3 days after irradiation for cell populations of the innate immune response and 7 days after irradiation for cell populations of the adaptive immune response). Excise the tumors and prepare single-cell suspensions for further antibody labeling of the desired surface or intracellular markers.

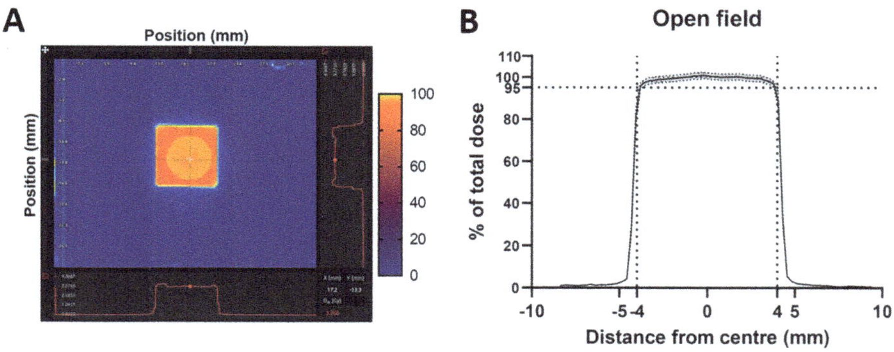

Fig. 3 Dose distribution with the 8 × 8 mm collimator. (**a**) 2D dose distribution using a tumor phantom with a diameter of 6 mm. Dose distribution was determined with an X-ray film. (**b**) 1D dose distribution within the 8 × 8 mm field

Acknowledgments

The authors acknowledge financial support from the Slovenian Research Agency under grant number P3-0003 and postgraduate research funding.

References

1. Lim JYH, Gerber SA, Murphy SP et al (2014) Type I interferons induced by radiation therapy mediate recruitment and effector function of CD8+ T cells. Cancer Immunol Immunother 63:259–271
2. Demaria S, Formenti SC (2012) Radiation as an immunological adjuvant: current evidence on dose and fractionation. Front Oncol 2:1–7
3. Heylmann D, Rödel F, Kindler T et al (2014) Radiation sensitivity of human and murine peripheral blood lymphocytes, stem and progenitor cells. Biochim Biophys Acta 1846:121–129
4. Bogdándi EN, Balogh A, Felgyinszki N et al (2010) Effects of low-dose radiation on the immune system of mice after total-body irradiation. Radiat Res 174:480–489
5. Billena C, Khan AJ (2019) A current review of spatial fractionation: back to the future? Int J Radiat Oncol Biol Phys 104:177–187
6. Yan W, Khan MK, Wu X et al (2019) Spatially fractionated radiation therapy: history, present and the future. Clin Transl Radiat Oncol 20: 30–38
7. Ha JK, Zhang G, Naqvi SA et al (2006) Feasibility of delivering grid therapy using a multileaf collimator. Med Phys 33:76–82
8. Wu X, Ahmed MM, Wright J et al (2010) On modern technical approaches of three-dimensional high-dose lattice radiotherapy (LRT). Cureus. https://doi.org/10.7759/cureus.9
9. Tubin S, Popper HH, Brcic L (2019) Novel stereotactic body radiation therapy (SBRT)-based partial tumor irradiation targeting hypoxic segment of bulky tumors (SBRT-PATHY): improvement of the radiotherapy outcome by exploiting the bystander and abscopal effects. Radiat Oncol 14. https://doi.org/10.1186/s13014-019-1227-y
10. Tubin S, Gupta S, Grusch M et al (2020) Shifting the immune-suppressive to predominant immune-stimulatory radiation effects by SBRT-PArtial Tumor Irradiation Targeting HYpoxic Segment (SBRT-PATHY). Cancers (Basel) 13:1–20
11. Fernandez-Palomo C, Fazzari J, Trappetti V et al (2020) Animal models in microbeam radiation therapy: a scoping review. Cancers 12. https://doi.org/10.3390/cancers12030527
12. Schültke E, Balosso J, Breslin T et al (2017) Microbeam radiation therapy – grid therapy and beyond: a clinical perspective. Br J Radiol 90:20170073. https://doi.org/10.1259/bjr.20170073
13. Markovsky E, Budhu S, Samstein RM et al (2019) An antitumor immune response is evoked by partial-volume single-dose radiation

in 2 murine models. Int J Radiat Oncol Biol Phys 103:697–708

14. Rivera JN, Kierski TM, Kasoji SK et al (2020) Conventional dose rate spatially-fractionated radiation therapy (SFRT) treatment response and its association with dosimetric parameters – a preclinical study in a Fischer 344 rat model. PLoS One 15:e0229053. https://doi.org/10.1371/journal.pone.0229053

Chapter 11

In Vivo Bioluminescence and Fluorescence Imaging: Optical Tool for Cancer Research

Duško Lainšček, Anja Golob-Urbanc, and Sara Orehek

Abstract

In vivo whole-body imaging, using optical tools based on bioluminescence and fluorescence detection, offers tremendous opportunities to specifically determine the spatiotemporal resolution of cancer cells within the tested animals. This enables the study of many aspects of cancer biology, including cell proliferation, trafficking, and invasions. The antitumor therapeutic properties of various tested compounds (e.g., CD19 CAR-T cells, used for cancer immunotherapy) can be monitored within the same animal at different time points, significantly reducing the number of animals used in the study as indicated in this method.

Key words Bioluminescence, Fluorescence, Photons, Luciferase, Substrates, Light absorption, Hemoglobin, Region of interest, Cancer, CAR-T cells

1 Introduction

Implementation of in vivo whole-body imaging, where observance of bioluminescence (BLI) or fluorescence is utilized, has brought tremendous advancement in biomedical research, where gene expression, protein–protein interaction, infections, and specific cell imaging can be investigated with a special emphasis on cancer research. Optical imaging allows monitoring of exogenously labeled cell proliferation, and trafficking, as well as determination of therapeutic properties of various administered cells and compounds. Bioluminescence and fluorescence detection in living organisms is safe, cost-effective, easy to use, and can be applied for studying various disease processes and biology in vivo. Cancer biology and antitumor therapy can be studied in a less invasive way that gives us a spatiotemporal-specific resolution of studied cells or substrates [1–4]. Despite BLI or fluorescence detection being very useful, there are some limitations and discrepancies that need to be considered. Compared to in vivo fluorescence, BLI has a low background and high sensitivity, making it very useful for the detection

Maja Čemažar, Tanja Jesenko and Urša Lampreht Tratar (eds.), *Mouse Models of Cancer: Methods and Protocols*, Methods in Molecular Biology, vol. 2773, https://doi.org/10.1007/978-1-0716-3714-2_11,
© The Author(s), under exclusive license to Springer Science+Business Media, LLC, part of Springer Nature 2024

of small cancer metastases or even specific cell trafficking (e.g., lymphocytes) [5–7]. On the other hand, deep tissue imaging is possible to some extent, whereas strong autofluorescence in the living organism hinders the detection of fluorescence in the deep tissue [1]. For fluorescence detection, an external light source should be provided which is not required for BLI imaging because it is based on the endogenous production of light triggered by the specific enzymatic activity of luciferase or analogs. Nonetheless, fluorescence detection takes only a few seconds, whereas BLI imaging usually takes more than a few minutes. However, BLI is more sensitive, meaning that smaller tumors can be visualized with higher sensitivity compared to fluorescently labeled cancer cells [5, 6, 8]. To produce luminescent signal specific substrates for enzymatic activity are needed [5]. The most commonly used luciferase is firefly luciferase (FLuc) derived from *Photinus pyralis.* Its specific substrate is luciferin and requires the addition of ATP, Mg^{2+}, and oxygen to emit a luminescent signal in the green spectrum with a maximum at 562 nm. Rluc from *Renilla reniformis* and Gluc from *Gaussia princeps* are frequently used ATP-independent enzymes with coelenterazine as substrate and maximum light emission at 480 nm as blue light [6, 9]. Furthermore, red light-emitting luciferases (e.g., click beetle luciferase) enhance BLI detection in deep tissue [6, 9, 10]. One of the drawbacks of BLI is luciferin's pharmacodynamic properties; it has a renal clearance of approximately 30 min, which means that repeated dosing for long-term visualization is required. In addition, blood-brain barrier (BBB) crossing is hampered for luciferin. To overcome these hurdles, Akaluc luciferase, a near-infrared emission that peaks at 677 nm was developed with Akalumine-hydrochloride as a specific substrate, which reportedly exhibits excellent BBB diffusion properties [11]. Although Akaluc was shown to be 100–1000 times more sensitive than FLuc, enabling real deep tissue visualization and improved imaging, some reports have pointed to possible toxicity of the substrate and high background signal within the liver [9]. What is more, the introduction of luciferases with various light-emitting properties enabled researchers to establish dual reporter systems like Akaluc-Antares luciferase pairs, which permit the tracking of differently labeled cancer cells [2, 12].

BLI has a drawback of some background signal; however, the occurrence of autofluorescence is a major problem in in vivo fluorescence detection as most endogenous fluorophores emit light in the range of blue-green spectrum which is strongly hindered by the high absorbance of hemoglobin and skin melanin [13, 14]. An optimal fluorescent label or probe for in vivo fluorescence imaging should have an emission maximum in the range of 650–900 nm, where the lowest light absorbance with less light scattering occurs. The usage of near-infrared (NIR) proteins, for instance iRFP [8, 13] allows deeper penetration and imaging (Fig. 1). Moreover,

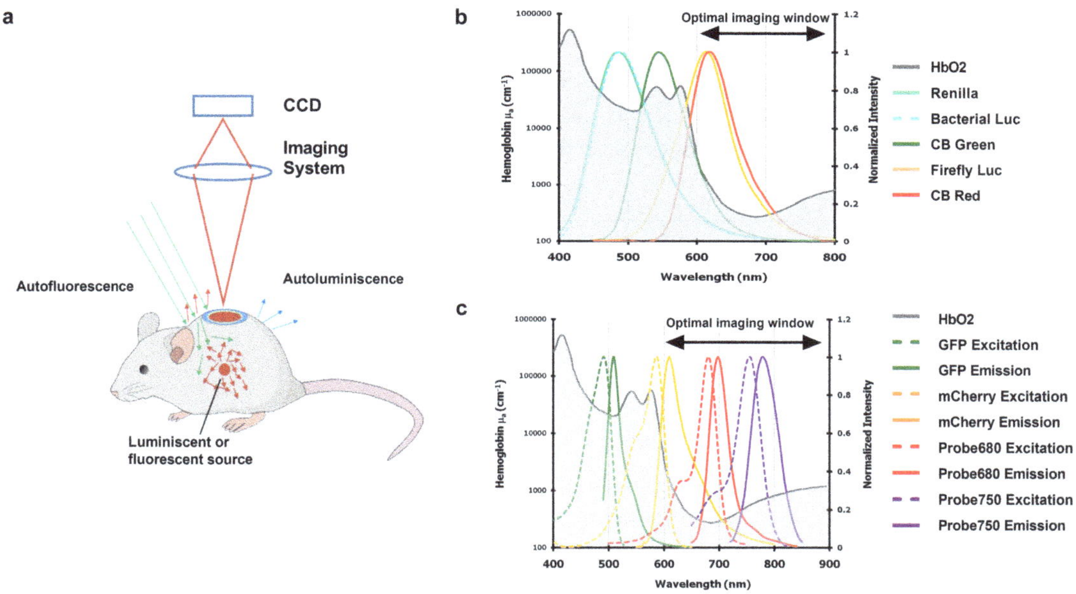

Fig. 1 Schematic presentation of IVIS system, used for bioluminescence or fluorescence imaging (**a**). Spectra of luciferase, used for BLI. Optimal luminescence imaging is from 600 to 800 nm (**b**). Spectra of fluorescent proteins or probes, used for fluorescence imaging. Fluorescent signal is higher than in BLI, but with lower sensitivity due to the high background. Optimal fluorescence imaging is from 620 to 900 nm (**c**). (Figure is reproduced with permission from PerkinElmer, Waltham, MA)

gastrointestinal content also hampers fluorescence detection due to high alfalfa and chlorophyll presence, a normal ingredient in most mouse chow. To reduce the autofluorescence in this part, special alfalfa-free diets can be fed to experimental mice [15].

As stated in vivo optical imaging is often used in cancer immunotherapy studies, investigating the efficacy of CAR-T cells. The chimeric antigen receptor (CAR) used in cancer therapy consists of an extracellular recognition domain (scFv), a hinge domain, a transmembrane domain, and cytosolic activation domains (CD28, CD137, or others, with CD3ζ) localized to the plasma membrane of T cells and is capable of recognizing tumor-specific surface molecules independently of the MHC. Upon specific recognition of tumor surface molecules, CAR-T cell activation occurs, leading to the killing of target cancer cells. Based on the success in several clinical trials, CD19 CAR-T cells were enlisted as an FDA-approved drug for treating B-cell leukemias and lymphomas [16–18]. With new variants of CAR-T cells (e.g., CAR-T cells targeting BCMA antigen, solid tumors, etc.) and other therapeutic cells emerging, in vivo imaging is indispensable in biomedical research.

Here, we describe the establishment of a mouse animal model to study the therapeutic properties of CD19 CAR-T cells. In vivo whole-body monitoring of the bioluminescence signal emitted by the target cancer Raji-FLuc cells (blood cancer model) allows us to monitor the killing of cancer cells throughout the time within the same animal, providing us with information about the immunotherapeutic state of the infused CD19 CAR-T cells. Additionally, imaging of the melanoma cancer model (solid cancer model) and in vivo fluorescence are described.

2 Materials

2.1 Cell-Associated Work

2.1.1 Equipment

1. Biosafety cabinet (class II, Type A or B).
2. Automated cell counter.
3. Centrifuge.
4. Humidified CO_2 incubator.
5. Ultracentrifuge (SW28 rotor).
6. SW32Ti Beckman rotor (or equivalent).
7. Inverted light microscope.
8. Benchtop centrifuge.
9. Flow cytometer.
10. Pipette gun.
11. P200 pipette (je posebaj omenjena v tekstu).
12. Thermoblock.
13. Water bath.

2.1.2 Reagents

1. Human embryonic kidney (HEK) 293T cells (ATTC).
2. Jurkat cell line (ATTC).
3. Raji-Burkitt's lymphoma B cells stably expressing FLuc (prepared in house or commercially available).
4. Human PBMCs (peripheral blood mononuclear cells), obtained from healthy volunteers.
5. Bioware® Brite B16F10-Red-FLuc (PerkinElmer).
6. Roswell Park Memorial Institute (RPMI) medium or RPMI-1640 medium.
7. Dulbecco's Modified Eagle's Medium (DMEM).
8. Heat-inactivated fetal bovine serum (FBS).
9. Phosphate buffered saline (PBS).
10. Trypsin-EDTA solution.
11. 0.4% Trypan blue solution.
12. T-75 tissue culture flask (treated for adherent cells and non-treated for suspension cells).
13. Conical tubes (15 mL and 50 mL; sterile).
14. 10 cm tissue culture treated dish.

15. Dimethyl sulfoxide (DMSO).
16. Plasmids: psPAX2 (Addgene Cat#12260); pMD2.G (Addgene Cat#12259), and a pLvx expression vector containing the gene for the second-generation chimeric antigen receptor anti-CD19 (with myc-tag) under EF1 alpha promoter (pLvx-CAR-CD19).
17. Polyethyleneimine (PEI), linear, MW 25,000.
18. 150 mM NaCl.
19. 50 mL syringe, sterile.
20. Ultracentrifuge tubes.
21. 0.45 μm pore size filter.
22. Tips with filter
23. 1.5 mL microtubes.
24. Flow cytometry tubes.
25. 24-well tissue culture plates.
26. Individually wrapped sterile serological pipettes.
27. Polybrene.
28. Isotype control: Mouse (E5Y6Q) mAb IgG2a Isotype Control (Alexa Fluor® 647 Conjugate) (Cell Signaling).
29. Antibody anti-myc: Myc-Tag (9B11) Mouse mAb (Alexa Fluor® 488 Conjugate) (Cell Signaling).
30. Ficoll-Paque density gradient media.
31. Pan T Cell Isolation Kit (Miltenyi).
32. ImmunoCult™ Human CD3/CD28/CD2 T Cell Activator (Stemcell Technologies, Inc.) or equivalent.
33. Human recombinant IL-2.
34. Parafilm.
35. Cryovial.

2.2 In Vivo Imaging

2.2.1 Equipment

1. Inhalation anesthesia system.
2. Heated surgical table.
3. IVIS® Lumina LT Series III Imaging system with integrated 150 Watt Tungsten/Halogen Lamp for fluorescence detection (PerkinElmer) or equivalent.
4. Living Image® 4.7.2 Software (PerkinElmer) or equivalent.
5. Mouse restrainer.

2.2.2 Reagents

1. D-Luciferin, Firefly, potassium salt, 1.0 g/vial.
2. Sterile phosphate buffer solution.
3. 0.2 μm filters.

4. 27 G needles, placed on 1 mL syringe.
5. 30 G insulin syringes.
6. 70% ethanol or any other disinfectant.
7. Isoflurane.
8. Eye ointment.
9. CD3-iRFP cells (prepared in house with transduction)
10. NSG (NOD.CB17-*Prkdc*^{scid} *IL2rg*^{tm1}*/BcgenHsd)* mice for xenograft cancer studies.
11. C57BL/6J OlaHsd mice for allogeneic cancer model.

3 Methods

Here, we describe a CD19 CAR-T cell preparation based on lentiviral transduction, used to treat the Raji-FLuc Burkitt's lymphoma cancer animal model. Labeled iRFP human T cells injection will be described as an in vivo fluorescence imaging model. For the xenograft cancer model, NGS mice lacking their own mature adaptive immune system are used [19], whereas C57BL/6J mice are used for the study of solid cancer. All animal experiments must be performed according to the national legislation upon obtaining an appropriate permit with emphasis on FELASA recommendations and 3R rule. Humane endpoints should be strictly established. The choice of whether to monitor bioluminescence or fluorescence signal depends on cancer cell labeling (e.g., cells, expressing luciferase or fluorescent proteins). All procedures on animals should be performed using minimal invasive approach, whereas injections should be administered aseptically and under general anesthesia offering supportive care, when appropriate.

3.1 General Maintenance of Cell Lines

Here we describe general guidance for the maintenance of adherent HEK293T cells, Bioware® Brite B16F10-Red-FLuc, and suspension cell lines (Raji and Jurkat). All protocols involving cells should be performed under sterile conditions in a laminar flow hood.

3.1.1 Adherent Cell Line (HEK293T, Bioware® Brite B16F10-Red-FLuc)

The HEK293T cell line is a derivative of the HEK293 cell line [19], commonly used as a lentiviral production cell line as it contains SV40 T-antigen which renders it more efficient for vector production [20]. Bioware® Brite B16F10-Red-FLuc is a mouse melanoma cell line that was stably transfected with the firefly luciferase gene from *Luciola Italica* (Red-FLuc).

1. Thaw the vial containing the cells in a 37 °C water bath or put the vial for 2 min to 37 °C preheated thermoblock.
2. Rapidly transfer thawed cells to a conical tube (15 mL) containing 10 mL of prewarmed DMEM supplemented with 10% FBS.

3. Centrifuge cells at 166× *g* for 5 min.
4. Discard the cell supernatant, resuspend the cell pellet in prewarmed 10 mL DMEM supplemented with 10% FBS, and transfer cell suspension to a T-75 flask.
5. Incubate the cells at 37 °C and 5% CO_2 in a humidified incubator and when they reach approximately 90% confluence, passage the cells.
6. Remove the spent culture media and wash cells with the 10 mL PBS (*see* **Note 1**).
7. Discard the PBS from the flask, add 2 mL of trypsin-EDTA solution and wait for 5 min for cells to detach from the flask surface.
8. Once detached, add 8–10 mL of DMEM supplemented with 10% FBS to inactivate the trypsin and transfer the cells into a conical tube (15 mL).
9. Centrifuge the cells at 166× *g* for 5 min.
10. Discard the supernatant and resuspend the cell pellet in 10 mL of DMEM supplemented with 10% FBS.
11. Dilute the sample of cell suspension in a 1:1 ratio (v/v) with trypan blue vital stain and count live (unstained) and dead (stained) cells using an automated cell counter.
12. For subculturing the cells seed them in a T-75 tissue culture flask at a concentration of 2–3 × 10^5 cells/mL in as many flasks as necessary (*see* **Note 2**) or follow Subheading 3.2, **step 1**, for plating cells for transfection (*see* **Note 3**).

3.1.2 Suspension Cell Line (Raji-FLuc and Jurkat)

1. Thaw the vial with the cells in a 37 °C water bath or put the vial for 2 min to 37 °C in a thermoblock.
2. Rapidly transfer thawed cells to a sterile conical tube (15 mL) containing 10 mL of prewarmed RPMI-1640 supplemented with 10% FBS.
3. Centrifuge the cells at 166× *g* for 5 min.
4. Discard the cell supernatant, resuspend the cell pellet in prewarmed 10 mL RPMI-1640 supplemented with 10% FBS, and transfer cell suspension to a T-75 flask.
5. Incubate the cells at 37 °C and 5% CO_2 in a humidified incubator and to passage the cells, change the media every 2–3 days or when the concentration of cells in the flask is 2–3 × 10^6 cells/mL (*see* **Note 3**).
6. Harvest the cells into a conical tube (15 mL) and centrifuge at 166× *g* for 5 min.
7. Discard the supernatant and resuspend the cell pellet in 10 mL of RPMI-1640 supplemented with 10% FBS.

8. Count the cells (*see* Subheading 3.1.1, **step 11**).
9. For subculturing the cells seed them in a T-75 tissue culture flask at a concentration of 1–3 × 10^5 cells/mL (*see* **Note 4**) in as many flasks as necessary.

3.2 Lentivirus Production

Here we describe a protocol for lentivirus production by transient transfection of HEK293T cells with a packaging plasmid, an envelope glycoprotein-encoding plasmid, and a lentiviral expression plasmid. Handling of lentiviral material is considered a biosafety level 2; therefore, all work should be performed in a sterile biosafety level 2 cabin in compliance with local biosafety rules and regulations.

1. Seed ten 10 cm culture dishes (*see* **Note 5**) with 5 × 10^6 HEK293T cells per dish in 10 mL DMEM supplemented with 10% FBS.
2. Incubate the cells overnight at 37 °C and 5% CO_2 in a humidified incubator to achieve approximately 60–80% confluency.
3. Prepare transfection mixture in two 15 mL conical tubes (amount for one 10 cm culture dish):
   - *Tube 1* (plasmid mixture): dilute the plasmids (12 μg psPAX2, 5 μg pMD2.G, and 15 μg of expression vector pLvx-CAR-CD19) in 150 mM NaCl to a total volume of 500 μL.
   - *Tube 2* (transfection reagent): Dilute PEI in 500 μL 150 mM NaCl. Generally, for 1 μg of plasmid mixture DNA, 6–12 μL of PEI solution will be required.
4. Pipette the solution from tube 2 to the solution in tube 1, vortex the conical tube, and incubate for 20–30 min at room temperature, then pipette the solution dropwise into the dish containing HEK293T cells. To evenly distribute the transfection mixture, gently swirl the dish back and forth.
5. Incubate the cells at 37 °C and 5% CO_2 in a humidified incubator overnight (approximately 18 h).
6. Replace the culture medium with fresh DMEM supplemented with 10% FBS, by slowly pipetting 10 mL per dish (*see* **Note 6**).
7. Incubate the cells for 48 h at 37 °C and 5% CO_2 in a humidified incubator (*see* **Note 7**).
8. Harvest the supernatant in a 50 mL conical tube.
9. Centrifuge the supernatant at 166× *g* for 5 min to pellet the cells and cell debris.
10. Filter the viral supernatant using a 50 mL syringe and 0.45 μm sterile filter and transfer it to an ultracentrifuge tube.

11. Balance the ultracentrifuge tubes to within 0.1 grams and centrifuge at 28,000 rpm (SW32Ti rotor) for 2 h at 4 °C.
12. Pour the supernatant from the ultracentrifuge tube into a waste bottle. While the ultracentrifuge tube is still inverted, remove the excess liquid with a P200 pipette (use tips with filter). The virus pellet should be visible at the bottom of the tube.
13. Add 100 μL RPMI-1640 to the ultracentrifuge tube, cover it with parafilm, and store it at 4 °C for 30 min to 1 h (or put it on ice for 15 min).
14. Resuspend the pellet by gently pipetting up and down multiple times and avoid bubble formation.
15. Aliquot the lentivirus solution into 1.5 mL microtubes and store at −80 °C (*see* **Note 8**).

3.3 Determination of Viral Titer by Flow Cytometry

Our CAR-CD19 design incorporates a myc tag between the signal peptide and scFv-CD19 to allow the detection of CAR receptor expression on the cell surface with an anti-myc antibody.

1. Seed 5×10^5 Jurkat cells in a 24-well tissue culture plate with a final volume of 400 μL per well (perform the experiment in duplicate).
2. Prepare working dilutions of lentivirus supernatants, for example 10×, 50×, and 250× in culture medium RPMI-1640.
3. Add 100 μL of each dilution to a well containing Jurkat cells to obtain 50×, 250×, and 1250× dilutions. Also include nontransduced cells where only 100 μL of culture medium is added.
4. Add polybrene to each well at a final concentration of 5 μg/mL.
5. After 48 h at 37 °C and 5% CO_2 in a humidified incubator, resuspend the cells in each well, count them and transfer at least 10^5 Jurkat cells into 1.5 mL microtubes.
6. Perform staining with the antibodies against myc tag according to the manufacturer's instructions (include the staining with isotype control and unstained Jurkat cells).
7. Analyze the cells by flow cytometry and quantify the percentage of myc-positive Jurkat cells.
8. To determine the lentivirus titer, use the following formula (*see* **Note 9**):

$$\mathrm{TU/mL} = (\text{number of cells transduced} \times \text{percent myc} - \text{positive cells} \times \text{dilution factor})/(\text{volume in mL per well}).$$

- If the 1250× dilution well has 20% myc-positive cells and 5×10^5 cells were originally transduced, then there are $(500{,}000 \times 0.25 \times 1250)/(0.5\ \mathrm{mL}) = 2.5 \times 10^8$ TU/mL.

3.4 Generation and Expansion of CAR-T Cells

3.4.1 Isolation of Human T Cells

1. Dilute the blood obtained from healthy donors with room temperature PBS in a 1:1 ratio (*see* **Note 10**).
2. Add 15 mL of Ficoll to a 50 mL conical tube.
3. With the gun pipet (use gravity delivery mode) gently layer the diluted blood over the Ficoll, avoiding disturbing the two layers.
4. Centrifuge 15 min at 950× *g* with brake off.
5. Transfer the cloudy layer (between the upper plasma and bottom Ficoll layer), containing the PBMC, to a 50 mL conical tube.
6. Wash the harvest cells twice with PBS (500× *g*, 10 min, brake on).
7. Resuspend the PBMCs in RPMI-1640 supplemented with 10% FBS.
8. Count cells (*see* Subheading 3.1.1, **step 11**) (*see* **Note 11**).
9. For the isolation of T cells use the Pan T Cell Isolation Kit (Miltenyi) and follow the manufacturer's instructions.

3.4.2 Transduction of Human T Cells

1. Adjust the concentration of isolated human primary T cells to 1×10^6 cells/mL in RPMI-1640 supplemented with 10% FBS and 50 IU/mL human recombinant IL-2.
2. Add 25 μL/mL ImmunoCult™ Human CD3/CD28/CD2 T Cell Activator to the cell suspension to activate the T cells.
3. After 48 h at 37 °C and 5% CO_2 in a humidified incubator examine the cells under the inverted light microscope to confirm cluster formation of cells.
4. Seed 1×10^6 activated T cells in a 24-well plate in 500 μL warm RPMI-1640 supplemented with 10% FBS and 50 IU/mL human recombinant IL-2.
5. Add lentivirus at a multiplicity of infection (MOI) 5–10. To calculate the volume of viral particles for a given MOI use the formula: (total number of cells seeded × desired MOI/viral titer in TU/mL). Viral titer is calculated when titrating lentiviruses on Jurkat cells (*see* Subheading 3.3, **step 8**).
6. Add polybrene to each well at a final concentration of 5 μg/mL.
7. Gently swirl the plate and incubate it in a humidified incubator at 37 °C and 5% CO_2 for 4 h.
8. Add 1 mL of prewarmed RPMI-1640 supplemented with 10% FBS and 50 IU/mL human recombinant IL-2 to each 24-well plate well.

3.4.3 Expansion of Human T Cells

1. Expand the transduced human T cells for up to 10–14 days.
2. Replace half of the medium (remove carefully without disturbing the cells) every 2 days and supplement it with IL-2 in a final concentration of 50 IU/mL.
3. Resuspend cells twice a week and count them (*see* Subheading 3.1.1, **step 11**). When cell density exceeds the concentration of 2×10^6 cells/mL, split the cells or transfer them to a larger format of well plates. Maintain the cells at a concentration of approximately 1×10^6 cells/mL.

3.4.4 Validation of CAR Expression

1. After the expansion of CAR-T cells, count the cells (*see* Subheading 3.1.1, **step 11**) and collect a sample of cell suspension for flow cytometric analysis (at least 10^5 cells per sample).
2. To determine the transduction efficiency, perform staining with antibodies against myc tag according to the manufacturer's instructions (include the staining with isotype control and unstained CAR-T cells) (*see* **Note 12**).
3. Analyze the cells by flow cytometry and quantify the percentage of myc-positive CAR-T cells.

3.5 Establishment of a Preclinical Cancer Model

3.5.1 CD19 CAR-T Cell Treatment for Burkitt's Lymphoma Animal Model

1. Place the NSG mouse in a mouse restrainer.
2. Obtain good lateral tail vein visualization (*see* **Note 13**).
3. Disinfect the tail with 70% ethanol and wait to dry off.
4. Inject 100 μL of PBS cell suspension with approximately $0.5–1 \times 10^6$ Raji-FLuc intravenously by using a 27 G needle injection (*see* **Note 14**).
5. Monitor animal well-being after the injection (approximately 2 h).
6. Approximately 4 days later determine the in vivo proliferation state of Raji-FLuc by monitoring the BLI (*see* Subheading 3.6.1); daily monitoring of animal body weight (*see* **Note 15**).
7. After the BLI is determined inject intravenously (lateral tail vein) 100 μL of PBS cell suspension with approximately $2.5–5 \times 10^6$ CD19 CAR-T cells intravenously by using 27 G needle injection (*see* **Notes 14** and **16**).
8. Determine the therapeutic properties of CD19 CAR-T cells at different time points by monitoring BLI (*see* Subheading 3.6.1) (Fig. 2).

3.5.2 Melanoma Solid Cancer Model

1. Place the C57BL/6J mouse in an isoflurane inhalation anesthesia chamber. For the induction of anesthesia use 1.5–1.7 MAC (Minimal Alveolar Concentration) and 1.2–1.5 MAC for maintenance.

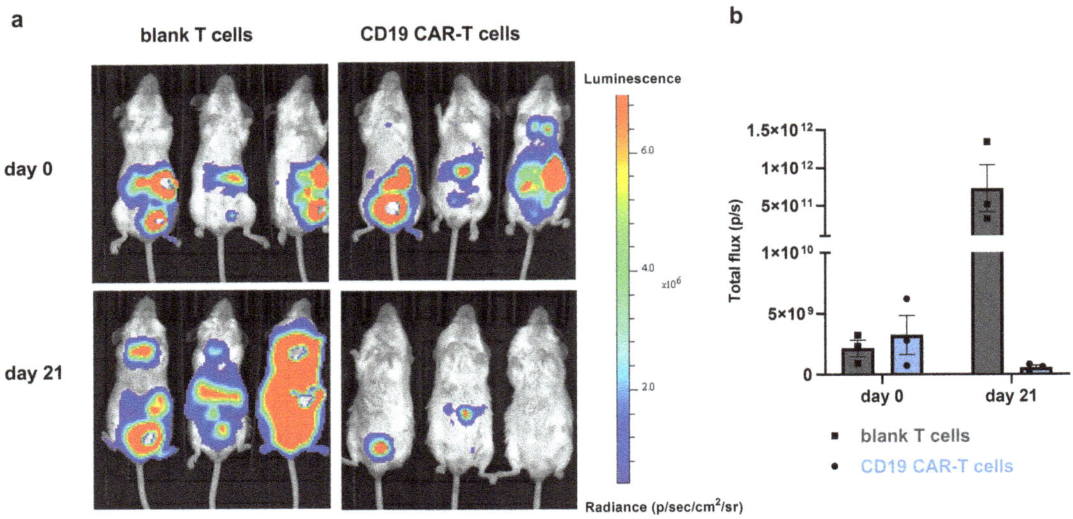

Fig. 2 Bioluminescence imaging determines CD19 CAR-T cell immunotherapeutic efficiency in NSG mice xenograft lymphoma cancer model (**a**). Graphic depiction of BLI measurements, presented in total flux of photons per second, measured in Living image 4.7.2 software (**b**)

2. Set the mouse on the heated surgical table under continuous inhalation anesthesia, remove the fur from the designated (right or left) flank of the animal, disinfect the area with 70% ethanol, and wait to dry it off.
3. Subcutaneously inject 150 μL of PBS cell suspension with 1×10^6 Bioware® Brite B16F10-Red-FLuc using a 27 G needle and monitor animal well-being after the injection.
4. Every 2 days, check the animal's body weight and tumor progression. When the tumor is palpable and reaches approximately 50 mm^3 (*see* **Note 17**), it is ready for further treatment. Additionally, monitor the BLI.

3.5.3 iRFP-Labeled CD3 Fluorescence Detection

1. Place the NSG mouse in a mouse restrainer.
2. Disinfect the abdomen region with 70% ethanol and wait to dry off.
3. Inject 100 μL of PBS cell suspension with approximately 1×10^6 CD3-iRFP cells (prepared in house with transduction) intraperitoneally by using a 27 G needle injection.
4. Monitor animal well-being after the injection (approximately 2 h).
5. Approximately 2 days later, determine the in vivo proliferation state of CD3-iRFP by monitoring the in vivo fluorescence (*see* Subheading 3.6.2).

3.6 In Vivo Imaging

Here, we describe the process of obtaining the whole-body in vivo luminescent or fluorescent signals, depending on the cell labeling. Bioluminescence imaging is explained for the Raji-FLuc lymphoma blood mouse model in NSG mice and the melanoma model in C57BL/6J mice. Fluorescence detection of human T cells, labeled with iRFP is shown in NSG mice. Imaging is performed under general anesthesia, using the IVIS Lumina LT Series III system with integrated Living Image software, but any other instrument capable of detecting BLI and fluorescence can be used.

3.6.1 Bioluminescence Imaging

1. Place the mouse, carrying FLuc cancer cells in an isoflurane inhalation anesthesia chamber. For induction use 1.5–1.7 MAK; for maintenance of anesthesia use 1.2–1.5 MAK.
2. Set the mouse on the heated surgical table with continuous inhalation anesthesia and apply the eye ointment to avoid cornea ulceration.
3. Prepare a stock solution of luciferin at 15 mg/mL in PBS. Filter sterilize through a 0.2 μm filter (*see* **Note 18**).
4. Inject luciferin subcutaneously at 150 mg luciferin/kg body weight 10–15 min before in vivo imaging (*see* **Note 19**).
5. Transfer the mouse into the IVIS in vivo imaging chamber connected to the inhalation anesthesia. The IVIS machine should be initialized before the imaging, resulting in cooling the CCD camera at −90 °C and heating the platform to 37 °C (green light stating readiness for imaging). Adjust the camera settings to obtain signal levels of 600–60,000 counts.
6. Adjust the settings: FOV to D, and check the luminescence and photography. Set binning to 8, and adjust the exposure time (e.g., 5 min). The emission filter should be open, and F/Stop is set to 1. The focus should be adjusted to the subject's height (1.5 cm) (*see* **Notes 20–23**). Autoexposure settings can also be used. Click Acquire to obtain the image.
7. Process the images. In the Units section, set the parameters to Counts or Radiance (photons/second) (*see* **Note 24**). Check the image min and max in the color scale to see if you are above the noise level or below CCD saturation. Additionally, there is a possibility to load a group of photos, where you can process them all at once (File-Browse-select folders).
8. To measure the signal click on the View-Tool Palette. Check Cosmic corrections to avoid artifacts in the Corrections section. In the Image Adjust section, you can change the Brightness, Contrast, and the Opacity of the image.

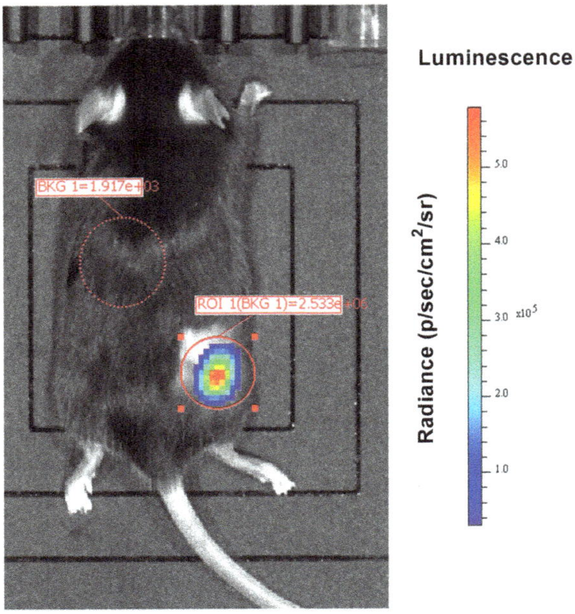

Fig. 3 ROI measurement in FLuc expressing melanoma model. First background signal (BKG1) was determined that was deducted in luminescent signal of solid cancer (ROI1 (BKG1))

9. In the Color scale section, determine the Limits factor on Auto. Choose the Color Table (e.g., Rainbow with Reverse depiction or with a Logarithmic Scale view of the color Table).
10. Determine the ROI (Region of interest). Draw a geometrical shape around your signal (e.g., square or circle). Name the ROI. Remove the background signal (*see* **Note 25**). Click on the Measure ROI (Fig. 3).
11. Obtain luminescent signal values that are either presented as a Total flux (photons/second) or as an Average Radiance (p/s/cm^2/sr). Image acquisition data is also obtained (e.g., Image overlay). Maximum radiance, Minimum radiance, and Stdev radiance values are also given by the measurement.

3.6.2 Fluorescence Imaging

1. Place the mouse, carrying FLuc cancer cells in an isoflurane inhalation anesthesia chamber. For induction use 1.5–1.7 MAK; for maintenance of anesthesia, use 1.2–1.5 MAK.
2. Set the mouse on the heated surgical table with continuous inhalation anesthesia and apply the eye ointment to avoid cornea ulceration.
3. Transfer the mouse into the IVIS in vivo imaging chamber connected to the inhalation anesthesia. The IVIS machine should be initialized before the imaging, resulting in cooling

the CCD camera at −90 °C and heating the platform at 37 °C (green light stating readiness for imaging). Turn on the Quartz Halogen Lamp.

4. Adjust the settings: FOV to D and check the Mode Fluorescent and Photograph. Set binning to 8, and adjust the exposure time first to Auto. Excitation and Emission filter should be open for the values depending on the fluorophore that we are monitoring (iRFP; Excitation 620–640 nm, Emission Cy 5.5. 670–710 nm). F/Stop is set to 2. The focus should be adjusted to the subject's height (1.5 cm). Check the Lamp Level to High. Click Acquire to obtain the image.

5. Process the images. In the Units section, set the parameters to Radiant Efficiency or Efficiency. In the Correction section, check Adaptive FL Background Subtraction. To determine the whole fluorophore spectra acquire the whole spectra by setting up the Imaging wizard (*see* **Notes 26** and **27**).

6. To compare different fluorescent signals (e.g., iRFP signal, tissue fluorescence, food fluorescence) to exclude a certain signal, perform the Spectral Unmixing (Fig. 4). In the Spectral Unmixing Section, check Automatic Method and then click Start Unmixing. Determine the Threshold on the Photograph. Select the two components (iRFP, Tissue Autofluorescence) that you want to unmix. PCA (Principle Component analysis) should be checked; the value should be approximately 100%. An alternative to spectral unmixing is Image Math (*see* **Note 28**).

7. Check the images and Radiant Efficiency where the sole iRFP signal of CD3-iRFP cells or Tissue Autofluorescence (AF) is presented. Unmixing results additionally in a composite image of iRFP and Tissue AF, depicted in different colors. By spectral unmixing, different fluorescent and bioluminescent reporters can be monitored at the same time (*see* **Note 29**).

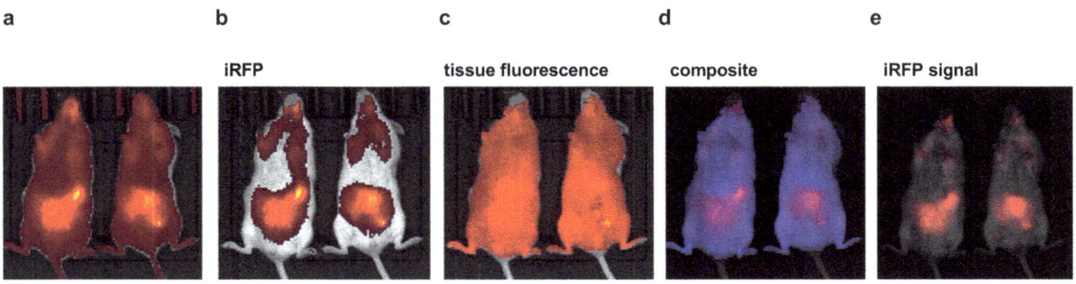

Fig. 4 In vivo fluorescent measurement of intravenously administered human T cells, labeled with iRFP (unmodified spectra) (**a**). Spectral unmixing was performed, considering iRFP (**b**) and tissue fluorescence (**c**) signal. Composite picture of iRFP and tissue fluorescence signal after spectral unmixing; blue color denoting tissue fluorescence, red color depicting iRFP fluorescence signal (**d**). Refined iRFP signal, depicting location of T cells in mice (**e**)

4 Notes

1. Carefully, without disturbing the cells, add PBS into the corner of the T-75 tissue culture flask to prevent the loss of the cells. Then gently swirl the flask for few times to wash the cells.
2. Subculture the cells every 2–3 days or when they reach approximately 90% confluence. Check the flask under an inverted light microscope every 24 h.
3. Human adherent and suspension cell lines should be expanded rapidly and stocks should be frozen in liquid nitrogen in a cryopreservation medium (FBS with 10% DMSO) at a low passage number. We usually freeze at approximately 2×10^6 cells per cryovial.
4. When subculturing the cells, we usually split cells every 2–3 days in a 1:10 ratio (discard 9 mL of cell suspension from the flask, leaving 1 mL of cell suspension, and add 9 mL of fresh culture media).
5. We are describing production in a volume of 100 mL, which usually results in virus stocks on the order of 1×10^8 transduction units (TU/mL). We prefer using 10 cm culture dishes but any format can be used.
6. The culture medium should be replaced with the fresh one after several hours posttransfection to remove the transfection mixture.
7. Lentiviruses should be harvested between 48 and 72 h after transfection when peak lentivirus production is reached; therefore, the supernatant may be harvested twice. First time 48 h after the transfection when the supernatant is replaced with the fresh medium and stored at 4 °C until the next day when it is combined with the second harvest of supernatant.
8. Frozen viruses are stable at −80 °C for up to 6 months. We recommend avoiding freeze-thaw cycles because with each cycle the lentivirus titer drops.
9. For accurate titration, use viral dilutions that give you 5–20% myc-positive cells, thus staying within the linear range. A higher percentage of myc-positive cells would result in an overestimation of the lentivirus titer, and therefore, the titers may not be reliable.
10. If the blood from a leukapheresis donor is used, blood dilution with a buffer of 1:3 or 1:4 is recommended. The collection of PBMCs from healthy volunteers should be permitted by the appointed national regulator.

11. PBMCs can be frozen in liquid nitrogen in a cryopreservation medium (FBS with 10% DMSO) at a concentration of approximately 5×10^6 cells/mL.
12. Transduction efficiency can also be determined during the expansion phase.
13. For a good lateral tail visualization provoke vasodilatation by placing the tail in a 40° water bath for 1 min.
14. Raji-FLuc cancer cells with subsequent injection of CD19 CAR-T cells can be also injected intraperitoneally.
15. The time, when BLI is monitored, can vary depending on the number of injected labeled cancer cells.
16. The number of injected CD19 CAR-T cells can differ, based on the effector:target ratio that we want to study.
17. 50 mm^3 is determined by using the volume formula $(\text{width} \times \text{length} \times \text{height} \times \pi)/6$.
18. Dissolved luciferin may be stored at 4 °C for up to 3 weeks; long-term storage at either 4 °C or −20 °C may result in a diminished BLI signal.
19. Luciferin can be administered also intraperitoneally, but 3–10% of injections can be given accidentally into the intestine [7].
20. FOV is determined by the distance between the lens and the sample. FOV A presents a 5 cm distance, FOV B 7.5 cm, FOV C 10 cm, and FOV D 12.5 cm. Some instruments have also FOV E (24 cm) and FOV Z (2.6 cm) options.
21. Exposure time is proportional to how long the light is collected through the open shutter. A shorter exposure time improves throughput and a longer exposure time increases intensity. Recommended maximum exposure time should be below 5 min.
22. F/Stop (Lens Aperture) determines the amount of light that is collected by the CCD camera. The maximum light collection is at F/Stop 1 (default settings for luminescence), whereas 16 (default settings for photo) is the smallest aperture, where we obtain the best resolution.
23. Binning gives the possibility to change sensitivity and resolution. It refers to grouping the pixels of the photo into a larger super-pixel. Large binning (set value 8) enables higher sensitivity with lower resolution, whereas small binning (value 2) offers lower sensitivity with higher resolution.
24. Value Counts is an uncalibrated measurement of the photon incident on the CCD camera. Proper image parameters should avoid image saturation and give a sufficient signal. The program will state when saturation occurs in red letters note. Radiance is a calibrated measurement of the photon emission

from the subject and is recommended for luminescent imaging. The radiance unit is photons/second/cm^2/steradian.

25. To determine the exact luminescent signal exclude the background noise levels. In the ROI Tools section, choose Average Bkg ROI in the Type section. Draw an ROI on the nonluminescent area and click Measure ROI. To exclude the background signal of ROI that you want to quantify, first draw an ROI around the luminescent signal. Also, an Auto FreeDraw is a possibility. Then click Measure ROI. After the measurement perform the right click and set Bkg ROI to BKG1 to get luminescent values without background noise. You can also measure the Distance values between two signal areas (Image X, Y; measure distance in cm between two or more ROIs).
26. Radiant Efficiency is a calibrated measurement and states a radiance per incident excitation power (μW/cm^2). To perform Adaptive FL Background Subtraction, you first set the Threshold on the image, where you want to do the subtraction.
27. Imaging wizard is used for sequence acquirement, meaning that the animal is imaged at different wavelength excitations with resulting different emissions. Mark excitations and emissions that you want to compare. Obtain the sequence. You can also alter the excitation length for each fluorophore. Additionally, you can set up a time series study, determining the time interval. Then perform spectral unmixing by choosing different fluorescence sources. As an alternative, you can use Overlaying Multiple Images. Click on the Tools-Image Overlay and then choose two images.
28. Image math is an alternative to spectral unmixing for removing the autofluorescence background signal from the image. Image math combines two images and mathematically creates a new image. In the Tools select Image Math and then choose two images that you want to combine. Image A is the primary image, whereas image B is the image with the background signal. Then click Compute "k" from ROI. To see the new image click Image display.
29. Spectral unmixing can be performed by using Auto Mode or by Manual Mode, where you individually choose the fluorophores that you want to compare.

Acknowledgments

This work was supported by Slovenian research agency program P4-0176, Slovenian research agency project J4-4563 to D.L., and a young researcher grant to S.O.

References

1. Imamura T, Saitou T, Kawakami R (2018) In vivo optical imaging of cancer cell function and tumor microenvironment. Cancer Sci 109: 912–918. https://doi.org/10.1111/cas.13544
2. Mezzanotte L, van 't Root M, Karatas H et al (2017) In vivo molecular bioluminescence imaging: new tools and applications. Trends Biotechnol 35:640–652. https://doi.org/10.1016/j.tibtech.2017.03.012
3. Tannous A, CEB and B (2011) Bioluminescence imaging: progress and applications. Trends Biotechnol 29:624–633. https://doi.org/10.1016/j.tibtech.2011.06.010.BIOLUMINESCENCE
4. Refaat A, Yap ML, Pietersz G et al (2022) In vivo fluorescence imaging: success in preclinical imaging paves the way for clinical applications. J Nanobiotechnol 20:1–22. https://doi.org/10.1186/s12951-022-01648-7
5. Choy G, O'Connor S, Diehn FE et al (2003) Comparison of noninvasive fluorescent and bioluminescent small animal optical imaging. Biotechniques 35:1022–1030. https://doi.org/10.2144/03355rr02
6. Close DM, Xu T, Sayler GS, Ripp S (2011) In vivo bioluminescent imaging (BLI): noninvasive visualization and interrogation of biological processes in living animals. Sensors 11:180–206. https://doi.org/10.3390/s110100180
7. Khalil AA, Jameson MJ, Broaddus WC et al (2013) Subcutaneous administration of D-luciferin is an effective alternative to intraperitoneal injection in bioluminescence imaging of xenograft tumors in nude mice. ISRN Mol Imaging 2013:1–7. https://doi.org/10.1155/2013/689279
8. Genevois C, Loiseau H, Couillaud F (2016) In vivo follow-up of brain tumor growth via bioluminescence imaging and fluorescence tomography. Int J Mol Sci 17. https://doi.org/10.3390/ijms17111815
9. Liu S, Su Y, Lin MZ, Ronald JA (2021) Brightening up biology: advances in luciferase systems for in vivo imaging. ACS Chem Biol 16: 2707–2718. https://doi.org/10.1021/acschembio.1c00549
10. Zambito G, Gaspar N, Ridwan Y et al (2020) Evaluating brightness and spectral properties of click beetle and firefly luciferases using luciferin analogues: identification of preferred pairings of luciferase and substrate for in vivo bioluminescence imaging. Mol Imaging Biol 22:1523–1531. https://doi.org/10.1007/s11307-020-01523-7
11. Iwano S, Sugiyama M, Hama H et al (2018) Single-cell bioluminescence imaging of deep tissue in freely moving animals. Science 80(939):935–939
12. Su Y, Walker JR, Park Y et al (2020) Novel NanoLuc substrates enable bright two-population bioluminescence imaging in animals. Nat Methods 17:852–860. https://doi.org/10.1038/s41592-020-0889-6
13. Filonov GS, Piatkevich KD, Ting LM et al (2011) Bright and stable near-infrared fluorescent protein for in vivo imaging. Nat Biotechnol 29:757–761. https://doi.org/10.1038/nbt.1918
14. Lifante J, Shen Y, Ximendes E et al (2020) The role of tissue fluorescence in in vivo optical bioimaging. J Appl Phys 128. https://doi.org/10.1063/5.0021854
15. Inoue Y, Izawa K, Kiryu S et al (2008) Diet and abdominal autofluorescence detected by in vivo fluorescence imaging of living mice. Mol Imaging 7:21–27. https://doi.org/10.2310/7290.2008.0003
16. Yoo HJ, Harapan BN (2021) Chimeric antigen receptor (CAR) immunotherapy: basic principles, current advances, and future prospects in neuro-oncology. Immunol Res 69:471–486. https://doi.org/10.1007/S12026-021-09236-X
17. Maude SL, Laetsch TW, Buechner J et al (2018) Tisagenlecleucel in children and young adults with B-cell lymphoblastic leukemia. N Engl J Med 378:439–448. https://doi.org/10.1056/NEJMOA1709866/SUPPL_FILE/NEJMOA1709866_DISCLOSURES.PDF
18. Xiao X, Huang S, Chen S et al (2021) Mechanisms of cytokine release syndrome and neurotoxicity of CAR T-cell therapy and associated prevention and management strategies. J Exp Clin Cancer Res 40:1–23. https://doi.org/10.1186/S13046-021-02148-6/TABLES/3
19. Dubridge RB, Tang P, Chao Hsia H et al (1987) Analysis of mutation in human cells by using an Epstein-Barr virus shuttle system. Mol Cell Biol 7:379–387. https://doi.org/10.1128/MCB.7.1.379-387.1987
20. Merten OW, Hebben M, Bovolenta C (2016) Production of lentiviral vectors. Mol Ther Methods Clin Dev 3:16017. https://doi.org/10.1038/MTM.2016.17

Chapter 12

Cancer Imaging by Intravital Microscopy: The Dorsal Window Chamber Model

Elisabeth Bellard and Muriel Golzio

Abstract

Intravital microscopy allows a direct visualization of cells' behavior in their environment in a living organism with all its complexity. With appropriated models, longitudinal studies of structural and functional changes can be followed in the same animal on long period. In the field of cancer, the dorsal window chamber model is the model of choice for tumor events such as cells migration, vessels growth, and their permeability or interactions between cells and vessels. Coupled with wide-field, confocal, or multiphoton fluorescence microscopes, high spatial and temporal resolutions of the cellular events can be analyzed in vivo.

Key words Intravital microscopy, Dorsal window chamber (DWC), Tumor angiogenesis, Cell tracking, In vivo imaging, Vascular permeability

1 Introduction

Elucidating the mechanisms of cancer initiation and progression is essential for the future development of effective therapies. Among the processes involved, tumor growth and invasion, angiogenesis, vascular and microenvironment remodeling, and immune infiltration have been explored by different approaches. A significant challenge to deeper understand these processes is having access to direct observation of events over time in a living animal.

Optical techniques have numerous advantages over other imaging modalities such as positron emission tomography (PET), magnetic resonance imaging (MRI), or computed tomography (CT). In fact, they allow low-cost experiments with numerous fluorescent sensors or reporter genes to explore various hypotheses with high spatial and temporal resolutions. Among these optical techniques, intravital microscopy techniques, and particularly the dorsal window chamber set-up, responded to this challenge, providing visualization of tissues with cellular and subcellular of resolution [1]. Today, the dorsal skinfold window chamber is one of the

Maja Čemažar, Tanja Jesenko and Urša Lampreht Tratar (eds.), *Mouse Models of Cancer: Methods and Protocols*, Methods in Molecular Biology, vol. 2773, https://doi.org/10.1007/978-1-0716-3714-2_12,
© The Author(s), under exclusive license to Springer Science+Business Media, LLC, part of Springer Nature 2024

most widely used intravital model for study of cancer invasion [2] and angiogenesis [3, 4].

This technique allows a direct visualization of tumor events, like cells migration, vessels growth, and permeability and interactions between cells and vessels [5]. To visualize cells, fluorescent protein expressing tumor cells or the use of transgenic mouse with specified fluorescent cells can be used [6]. To follow cells in the blood stream, fluorescently labeled cells (immune cells, red blood cells) can be intravenously injected [7]. To highlight vessels, plasmatic markers (labeled fluorescent dextrans) or lectins targeting the vessels wall can be injected intravenously [8].

For imaging, the use of an upright macroscope or videomicroscope offers a large working space and long working distance objectives, ideal for optimal mice positioning [9]. A videomicroscope offers a large working space and allows acquisitions at video rate [10]. The use of a multiphoton microscope allows the visualization of the 3D tissue in depth with a high spatial resolution in *x*, *y*, and *z* axes [6–8].

Here, we described the surgical procedure for beginners and some illustrations related to vasculature observation in macroscopy and multiphoton microscopy.

2 Materials

2.1 Mice, Analgesia, and Anesthesia

1. Mice (*see* **Note 1**).
2. 0.3 mg/mL buprenorphine for analgesia.
3. 100 mg/mL ketamine for anesthesia.
4. 2 g/100 mL xylazine for sedation.
5. 0.9 % chloride sodium (NaCl).

2.2 Reagents and Equipment for Mice Surgery

2.2.1 Reagents for Mice Preparation and Surgical Area Preparation

1. Betadine for skin asepsis.
2. Depilatory cream for hair removal.
3. Ocular gel to protect the eyes.
4. 70% Ethanol.
5. Anios Spray.

2.2.2 Equipment for Mice Preparation

1. Sterile cotton gauze ×2.
2. Electric shaver for mice.
3. Sterile surgical drape.
4. Stem.
5. 0.3 and 0.5 mL syringes, 29 G needles.
6. Syringes 1 mL.

7. 50 mL Falcon tube and rack for 50 mL tube.
8. 1 mL Eppendorf tubes.
9. Heated red lamp.
10. LED lamp magnifier.
11. Glass-bead sterilizer.
12. Nitrile surgical gloves.
13. Surgical facemask.

2.3 Equipment Specific for Dorsal Window Chamber Surgery

1. Flat bag for steam sterilization of all metallic and glass items.
2. Window chamber kit: two symmetrical titanium frames with stainless steel screws, nuts, and retaining ring (APJ Trading Co., Ventura, CA, US) (Fig. 1A).
3. Sterile glass coverslip, 12 mm diameter (Ted Pella).
4. 35 mm Petri dish.
5. Sterile 5.0 silk suture with Cutting 3/8 Circle Needles (Peters Surgical, France).
6. Two sterile 100 mm Polystyrene petri dishes.
7. Specific surgical instruments (Fig. 1B):
   - Micro-Mosquito Hemostat Angled 90° for retaining ring positioning (FST) (Fig. 1B, a).
   - Fine Iris Scissors straight (FST) (Fig. 1B, b).
   - Dumont #4 forceps (Fig. 1B, c).
   - Halsey needle holder (FST) (Fig. 1B, d).
   - Bulldog clamps (straight) (Fig. 1B, e).
   - Noyes Spring Scissors (curved) for skin removal (Fig. 1B, f).
   - Extra Fine Graefe Forceps (curved) for skin removal (FST) (Fig. 1B, g).
   - S&T SuperGrip Forceps (JF-5TC – Angled 45°) for fat and connective tissue removing (FST) (Fig. 1B, h).
   - Moria Miniature Vannas Spring Scissors-Straight or curved for fat and connective tissue removing (FST) (Fig. 1B, i).
8. Others instruments: Socket wrench and Hole Punch Plier 1.0 mm (Fig. 1C).
9. Dissection microscope (Leica MZ FLIII) with a cold light source (KL 1500 LCD, Schott).

2.4 Equipment for Tumor Implantation

Modified glass 25 μL volume microsyringe with 29 G needle (Hamilton Company) for injection of tumor cells.

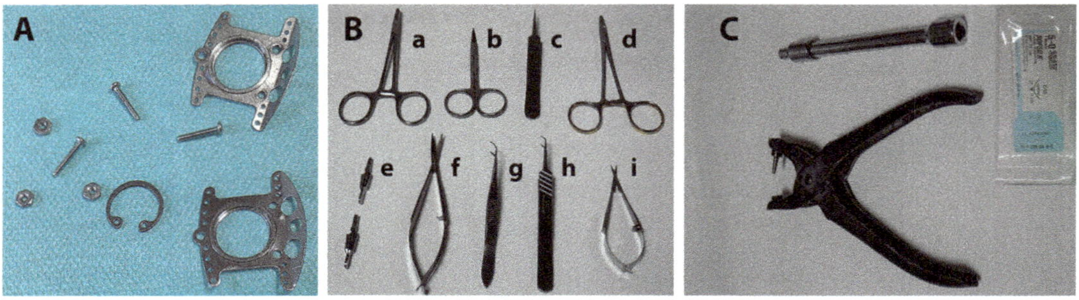

Fig. 1 Equipment for dorsal window chamber. (**A**) Window chamber kit is composed by two symmetrical titanium frames with stainless steel screws, nuts, and retaining ring. (**B**) Surgical instruments (scissors, forceps, and clamps). (**C**) Other instruments (wrench and punch)

2.5 Reagents and Equipment for Mice Imaging

1. Anesthesia-specific reagents and equipment:
   - Isoflurane (Vetflurane, Virbac).
   - Oxygen concentrator (Taema, TEM-SEGA).
   - Mask (Mini-Hub, TEM-SEGA).
2. Environment-Specific Equipment
   - 37 °C heating pad (mTCII micro-Temp Controller, Cell MicroControls).
   - 31 °C heating chamber.

2.6 Imaging-Specific Equipment

According to imaging modality:

- Upright macroscope (LEICA Macrofluo).
- Videomicroscope (LEICA DM6FS).
- CCD or SCMOS camera.
- Upright multiphoton microscope (Zeiss 7MP).
- Tunable Ti-Sapphire femtosecond laser, Chameleon Vision 2 (Coherent Inc.).
- Imaging support.

3 Methods

3.1 Instruments Preparation and Sterilization

All items necessary for surgery have to be sterilized before surgery: window chamber kit, Micro-Mosquito Hemostat, fine Iris Scissors, Dumont #4 forceps, Noyes Spring Scissors, Extra Fine Graefe Forceps, S&T SuperGrip Forceps, Miniature Vannas Spring Scissors, Halsey needle holder, Bulldog clamps, hole Punch Plier, socket wrench, and petri dish with glass coverslips inside.

1. Place all items in flat bags for steam sterilization.
2. Use one flat bag per window chamber kit, one for instruments, one for the hole punch plier and the socket wrench, and a last one for glass coverslips placed in the glass petri dish.
3. Autoclave all items for 20 min at 121 °C.

3.2 Preparation of the Solutions and Cells

Prepare all solutions under a laminar flow HEPA-filtered hood to keep them sterile.

1. Prepare buprenorphine solution for the number of mice planned +1 by diluting 0.3 mg/mL stock solution at a final concentration of 20 μg/mL for a subcutaneous injection at 0.1 mg/kg (~100 μL per 20 g mouse). For this, sample Buprenorphine with a 0.3 mL syringe and complete with suitable volume of sterile NaCl 0.9% in a 1 mL Eppendorf tube (*see* **Note 2**).
2. Prepare the mix of Ketamine and Xylazine for the number of mice planned +1 by sampling volumes appropriate for a 150 μL intraperitoneal injection at 100 mg/kg of Ketamine and 20 mg/kg of Xylazine, diluted in sterile NaCl 0.9% (*see* **Note 3**).
3. Prepare tumor cells suspension by suspending the cultured cells in NaCl 0.9% at a concentration providing 3×10^5 cells for a volume of 5 μL for injection (*see* **Note 4**).

3.3 Surgical and Dissection Areas Preparation

Window chamber surgery must be performed as sterile as possible to minimize the risk of animal infection. Before surgery, spray all surfaces before depilation and before surgery with Anios to clean and wipe it, particularly the stem placed in the middle of the surgical area and the lamp magnifier placed just behind the stem to illuminate the surgery area (Fig. 2a).

1. Place the glass-bead sterilizer in an accessible location closed to surgery area and switch on it.
2. Place the heated red lamp above the surgery area oriented so as to warm the mouse during the procedure.
3. Cover surgical and dissection area with the sterile surgical drape without touching the surface of the drape to provide a broad sterile surface for surgery and dissection (Fig. 2a). Once installed, carefully unwrap and drop the sterile cotton gauzes, prepackaged instruments, sterile suture threads, and window chamber kit on the sterile surgery and dissection areas without touching it.
4. Place the two sterile Petri dishes in a laminar flow HEPA-filtered hood to fill them with sterile NaCl 0.9% and 70% EtOH respectively and position them on one side of the sterile surgical drape.

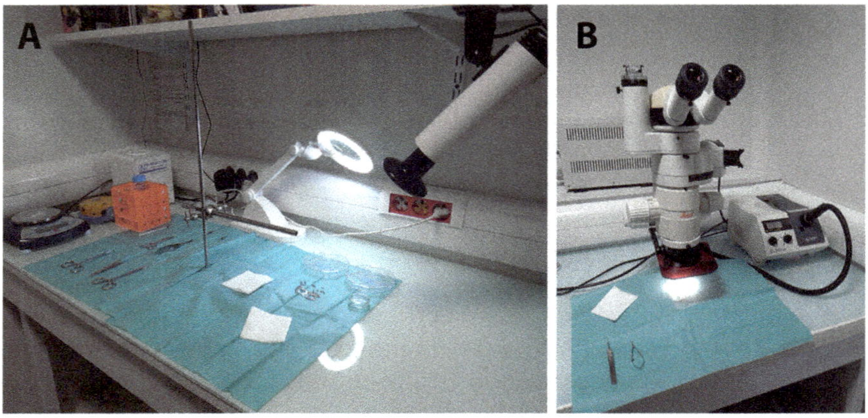

Fig. 2 Surgical and dissection areas preparation. (**a**) Surgical area and (**b**) dissection area

5. In the same way, place a 50 mL Falcon tube on a rack, fill it with sterile NaCl 0.9% and position it on one side of the sterile surgical drape with a sterile 1 mL syringe (Fig. 2a).
6. After cleaning and wiping with Anios, position the betadine and ocular gel on the sterile surgical drape.

3.4 Surgery Procedure

1. Thirty minutes before surgery, use 0.3 mL Micro-Fine syringe to inject subcutaneously the mouse with 0.1 mg/kg of the prepared Buprenorphine solution for pain management.
2. On a separate area dedicated to anesthesia and shearing, anesthetize the mouse by intraperitoneal injection, with a 0.5 mL Micro-Fine syringe, of the ketamine/xylazine solution.
3. For mice with hair, use the electric shaver to shear the dorsal area from the nape of the neck to the base of the tail along the back and on each side. Apply depilatory cream on the shorn area during less than 1 min and rinse with temperate water (*see* **Note 5**).
4. Transfer mouse to surgery area, just below the stem, on one sterile cotton gauze.
5. Apply ocular gel on the mouse's eyes to maintain hydration.
6. Apply two times betadine solution to the back of the mouse and the tail with cotton gauze.
7. Use the lamp magnifier to transilluminate the skinfold and suspend the mouse to the stem with two suture threads positioned on each side of the future chamber so as to have symmetrical patterns of blood vessels on each side of the dorsal midline align. Maintain the suture threads to the stem using the two bulldog clamps (Fig. 3a).
8. Place one of the two window chamber frames behind and against the skinfold, just between the two attachment points

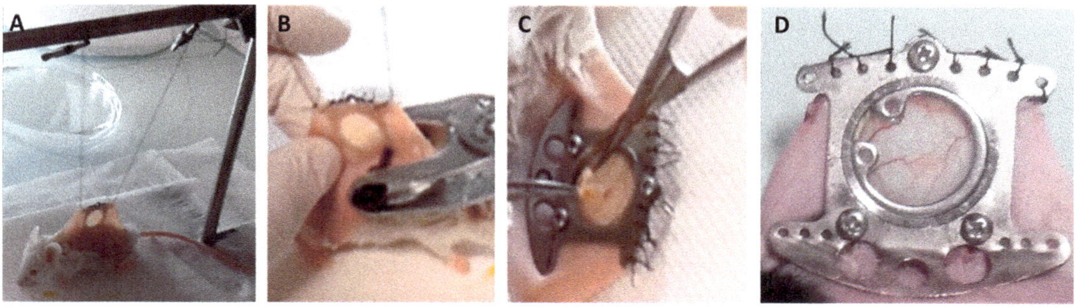

Fig. 3 Surgical and dissection procedure. (**a**) Illustration for **step 7**, (**b**) illustration for **step 9**, (**c**) illustration for **step 10**, and (**d**) illustration for **step 13**

of suture threads suspending the mouse, and suture the frame to the skin with six stitches on eight small holes available along the edge of the frame, leaving the penultimate free on each side. This side of the frame is the one that will be cut to remove the forward-facing portion of skin. Between uses of suture threads, place it in EtOH petri dish and rinse it in NaCl 0.9% petri dish before re use.

9. Punch two holes in the skin through both sides of the window chamber where the screws have to be positioned using the hole punch plier (Fig. 3b). Place the second frame in front of the skinfold, position the three screws and fasten them with nuts and the socket wrench so as to hold both frames together without tightening them too much to avoid circulation inhibition which could lead to necrosis. Suture the two frames to the skin with two stitches in the two remaining small holes along the edge of the frames.
10. Detach the mouse from the stem and position it on the side, facing to cut on top. Using Spring scissors and extra fine Graefe forceps, cut along the circumference of the internal window area and remove the forward-facing portion of skin leaving the opposite layer intact. Ensure that the cut area is fully sealed by the two frames (Fig. 3c).
11. Move the mouse to the dissection microscope and with Super-Grip forceps and miniature Vannas Spring scissors, remove remaining fat and connective tissue leaving intact the fine fascial plane covering dermis.
12. Using the modified glass microsyringe with 29 G needle with the bevel up and with a reduced angle, inject ~5 μL of the vortexed tumor cell suspension between the exposed fascial plane and the dermis. A small bubble should be visible.
13. With 1 mL syringe, fill the window with NaCl 0.9%, place the glass cover slip over the window and secure it with the retaining

ring using the micro-mosquito hemostat Angled 90°. Ensure that no air bubbles remain within the sealed window (Fig. 3d).

14. Return the mouse to the cage for recovery.
15. For further surgeries, wipe down and resterilize the contaminated surgical instruments with the glass-bead sterilizer.

3.5 Animal Housing and Recovery

1. Return the mouse to the animal housing facility after it has fully recovered from anesthesia (after ~1 h). House animals in conventional type 2 cages with only one individual per cage to prevent them from injuring each other.
2. The observation of animals after surgery should be daily, according to appropriate guidelines for pain management and limit points, checking for general appearance, weight, posture, and facial expression.
3. The appearance of the chamber is also controlled for inflammation or infection, and if limit points are met, experiment should be stopped.
4. Tumor growth should be visually apparent within 4–5 days and can be followed up to 15 days (Fig. 4).

3.6 Imaging

Use Isoflurane for anesthesia during imaging sessions. To allow acquisition on long term period in the same animal, couple microscopes with an anesthesia device, an oxygen concentrator, and a mask as well as with a 37 °C heating pad or 31 °C heating chamber according to the device.

3.6.1 Wide-Field Microscopy

Use an upright macroscope or videomicroscope with suitable light source and filter cubes coupled to a cooled CCD or sCMOS camera. A macroscope offers a large working space and long working distance objectives, ideal for optimal mice positioning. A videomicroscope offers a large working space when equipped with a Gibraltar platform and allows acquisitions at video rate in one color. When equipped with a beam splitter (Gemini, Hamamatsu), it can acquire simultaneously two colors at a high speed.

3.6.2 Multiphoton Microscopy

Use an upright microscope with suitable non-descanned detectors and filter cubes coupled to a tunable Ti-Sapphire femtosecond laser. Multiphoton microscopy allows the visualization of 3D tissue in depth (200 μm) with a spatial resolution of 300 nm in x and y axes and 2 μm in z axis.

Imaging device consists in a custom-made stiff plastic support (2–3 mm thick) with three small holes drilled in it at the position of screws and a 12 mm hole in the middle for access to imaging area. Threw nuts will allow to fix the window chamber to this support. This imaging support will be fixed to two others plastic support (5 mm thick) with double-sided tape, the two supports itself fix by

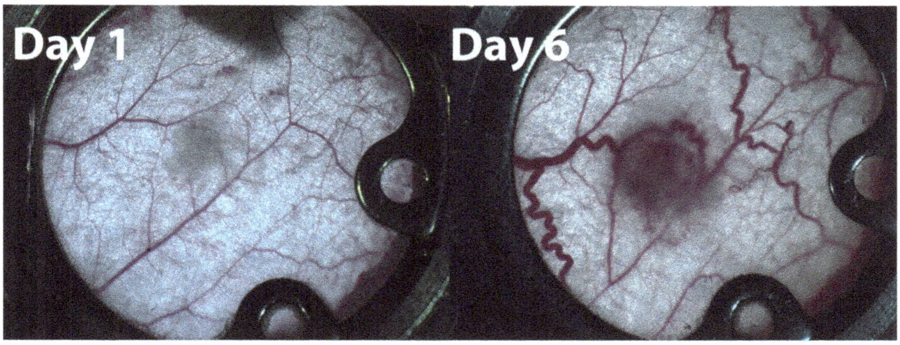

Fig. 4 Pictures of a tumor after surgery. Dorsal window chamber containing a tumor of B16F10 melanoma observed by brightfield macroscopy (without zoom) at day 1 and day 6

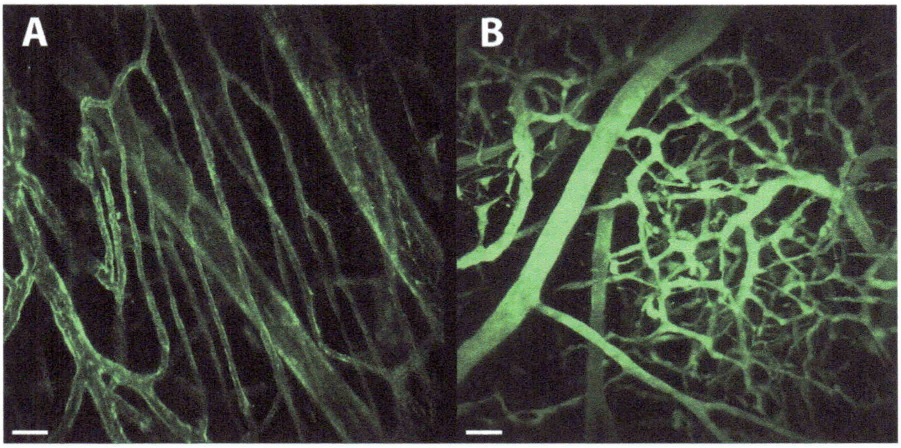

Fig. 5 Architecture of blood vessels revealed by fluorescent dextran (FD20) intravenous injection and observed by macrofluorescence microscopy. (**a**) Organized normal vessels and (**b**) disorganized tumor vessels. Scale bar = 50 μm

the same way to an overstage suitable for the microscope stage. The window chamber has to stay fixed on the imaging device to avoid motion artifacts during imaging sessions.

1. Turn on microscope, fluorescence source, camera, heating device, and anesthesia systems.
2. Anesthetize the mouse by placing it in an induction chamber with 2% volume isoflurane, and once unconscious, transfer it to a mask while attaching the mouse to the imaging device.
3. Clean the glass window with a cotton swab soaked in alcohol and protect mouse eyes with ocular gel.
4. Once attached, transfer the mouse and its support on the microscope stage and place its muzzle in the anesthesia mask with 1% isoflurane.

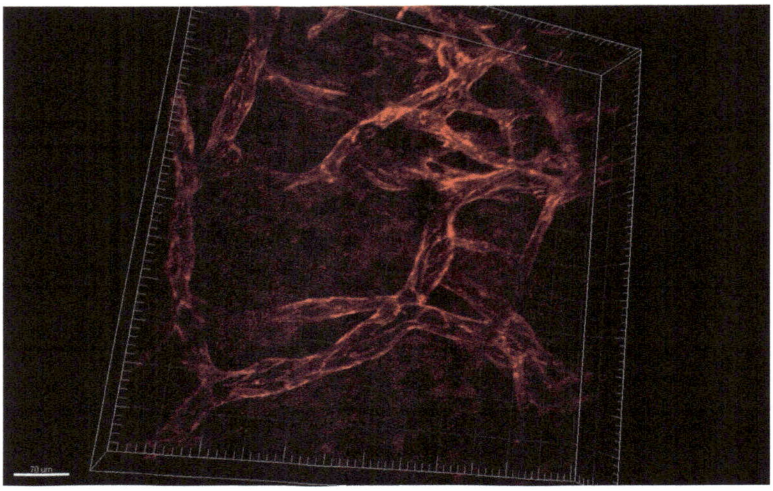

Fig. 6 In vivo visualization of endothelial cells in tumor. Architecture of tumor blood vessels revealed by intravenous injection of rat anti-mouse CD31 Alexa 647 antibody and observed by multiphoton microscopy. Scale bar = 70 μm

5. For fluorescence imaging select, the objective, the filter cube suitable for the fluorophore to image and, in case of multiphoton imaging, the appropriate wavelength for excitation.
6. To highlight vessels, inject intravenously plasmatic marker (labeled dextran) or lectins to target the vessels wall (Fig. 5). To target endothelial cells, inject intravenously labeled CD31 antibody 4 h before imaging session (Fig. 6).
7. To follow cells, you can inject it in intraorbital or intravenously or use transgenic mouse with specified fluorescent cells.
8. To acquire a wide-field sequence of images (time-lapse), adjust the focus and define the exposure time for each fluorophore such as not saturating the camera.
9. To acquire a multiphoton sequence of images, define the laser power such as not alter the tissue and adjust the detectors amplification gain and offset to optimize signal for each fluorophore. To obtain a stack of images in *Z* at each time point, define the top and bottom and the *Z* axial resolution (*see* **Note 6**).

4 Notes

1. Dorsal window chamber surgery can be performed on a wide variety of mouse strains. User just has to ensure that the mouse strain is compatible with the tumor cell line to study. All animal experiments have to be conducted in accordance with

procedural guidelines for animal handling and with approval from the Ethical Review Committee.

2. Buprenorphine has an expiration date and can be stored at room temperature in a safety deposit box.
3. Do not prepare the mix in advance. Ketamine and Xylazine have an expiration date and can be stored at room temperature in a safety deposit box.
4. Suspended cells should be used the day of surgery.
5. For surgery on hairless mice, proceed directly to next step.
6. During acquisition take attention not to have *Z* drift to maintain the same acquisition zone all along the acquisition time.

Acknowledgments

We thank Dr. Philippe Guy and Dr. Véronique LeCabec for the acquisition of the pictures of Fig. 3, Dr. Sophie Chabot for Fig. 4, Dr. Sandrine Pelofy for Fig. 5, and Dr. Bostjan Markelc for Fig. 6. We acknowledge the IPBS Genotoul core facilities, ANEXPLO and TRI, member of the national infrastructure France-BioImaging supported by the French National Research Agency (ANR-10-INBS-04).

References

1. Ellenbroek SIJ, van Rheenen J (2014) Imaging hallmarks of cancer in living mice. Nat Rev Cancer 14:406–418. https://doi.org/10.1038/nrc3742
2. Makale M (2007) Intravital imaging and cell invasion. Methods Enzymol 426:375–401. https://doi.org/10.1016/S0076-6879(07)26016-1
3. Jain RK, Munn LL, Fukumura D (2002) Dissecting tumour pathophysiology using intravital microscopy. Nat Rev Cancer 2:266–276. https://doi.org/10.1038/nrc778
4. Makale M (2008) Chapter 8. Noninvasive imaging of blood vessels. Methods Enzymol 444:175–199. https://doi.org/10.1016/S0076-6879(08)02808-5
5. Beerling E, Ritsma L, Vrisekoop N et al (2011) Intravital microscopy: new insights into metastasis of tumors. J Cell Sci 124:299–310. https://doi.org/10.1242/jcs.072728
6. Gui P, Ben-Neji M, Belozertseva E et al (2018) The protease-dependent mesenchymal migration of tumor-associated macrophages as a target in cancer immunotherapy. Cancer Immunol Res 6:1337–1351. https://doi.org/10.1158/2326-6066.CIR-17-0746
7. Asrir A, Tardiveau C, Coudert J et al (2022) Tumor-associated high endothelial venules mediate lymphocyte entry into tumors and predict response to PD-1 plus CTLA-4 combination immunotherapy. Cancer Cell 40:318–334.e9. https://doi.org/10.1016/j.ccell.2022.01.002
8. Markelc B, Bellard E, Sersa G et al (2018) Increased permeability of blood vessels after reversible electroporation is facilitated by alterations in endothelial cell-to-cell junctions. J Control Release 276:30–41. https://doi.org/10.1016/j.jconrel.2018.02.032
9. Bellard E, Markelc B, Pelofy S et al (2012) Intravital microscopy at the single vessel level brings new insights of vascular modification mechanisms induced by electropermeabilization. J Control Release 163:396–403. https://doi.org/10.1016/j.jconrel.2012.09.010
10. Carrière V, Colisson R, Jiguet-Jiglaire C et al (2005) Cancer cells regulate lymphocyte recruitment and leukocyte-endothelium interactions in the tumor-draining lymph node. Cancer Res 65:11639–11648. https://doi.org/10.1158/0008-5472.CAN-05-1190

Chapter 13

Imaging of Extravasation of Splenocytes in the Dorsal Skinfold Window Chamber

Tim Bozic and Bostjan Markelc

Abstract

Infiltration of immune cells into the tumor is one of the major drivers of antitumor immune response, which can direct the outcome of anticancer therapies. In mice, implantation of dorsal skinfold window chamber (DSWC) combined with intravital confocal fluorescence microscopy allows real-time observation of splenocyte extravasation and infiltration into tumors. Here, we describe a detailed procedure of the DSWC implantation, splenocyte isolation and fluorescent labeling, intravenous injection of labeled splenocytes, and imaging of splenocyte extravasation into tumors using confocal fluorescence microscopy.

Key words Splenocyte extravasation, Dorsal skinfold window chamber (DSWC), Intravital imaging, Fluorescence confocal microscopy

1 Introduction

Tumor immune cell infiltrate that differs between tumor types is emerging as an important immunostimulatory efficacy indicator of anticancer therapies. Increased infiltration of effector or regulatory immune cells into tumors corresponds to distinct tumor immune response signatures, which indicates proinflammatory or immunosuppressive tumor microenvironment [1]. In different cancers, the number of specific subsets of tumor-infiltrating immune cells and the susceptibility of cancer cells to different immune responses are key prognostic parameters [2]. Understanding how different therapies affect the infiltration of immune cells into tumors can help identify new potential targets and develop successful anticancer therapy [3]. In addition to the different subtypes of infiltrated immune cells and their localization, the fate of immune cells in the tumor microenvironment plays a key role in a sustained and efficient tumor immune response and in the development of immune memory [4, 5]. Therefore, methods that allow investigation of the complex nature of tumor-infiltrating immune cells are

Maja Čemažar, Tanja Jesenko and Urša Lampreht Tratar (eds.), *Mouse Models of Cancer: Methods and Protocols*, Methods in Molecular Biology, vol. 2773, https://doi.org/10.1007/978-1-0716-3714-2_13,
© The Author(s), under exclusive license to Springer Science+Business Media, LLC, part of Springer Nature 2024

essential for determining therapeutic efficacy and outcome [6–8]. Although flow cytometry, immunohistochemistry, gene expression, and other methods represent adequate techniques which can provide quantitative and spatial data, the temporal dynamics of migrating cells and their retention in the tumor are often overlooked [9]. On the other hand, the dorsal skinfold window chamber (DSWC) in mice allows the observation of living tissues, including tumors, which can be followed over a continuous period of time (up to 3 weeks). In addition to tumor models, the applications of DSWC extend to studies of tumor–stroma interaction [10], tumor-induced angiogenesis [11], and tumor response to treatments such as vascular-targeting agents [12–15], nanoparticles [16], siRNA [17], and radiotherapy [18, 19]. Although the first use of the DSWC model was reported many years ago, the development of novel imaging techniques, fluorescent proteins and probes [20, 21], and transgenic mouse models [22] has allowed the observation of molecular structures at higher resolution. The DSWC model is therefore particularly well suited for studies of vascular network and immune cell migration, since it enables examination of cells and structures with sufficient resolution when combined with fluorescence microscopy [23]. Here we describe in detail intravital imaging of extravasation of fluorescently labeled splenocytes into murine tumors growing in the DSWC model.

2 Materials

2.1 Implantation of the Dorsal Skinfold Window Chamber (DSWC)

1. Mice (Balb/c, weighing 18–22 g).
2. Disinfectant.
3. Suitable operating room equipped with HEPA filtered ventilation system.
4. Titanium window chamber set (Small Dorsal Kit, APJ Trading).
5. Stainless steel surgical tools.
    (a) Pean forceps (MicroMosquito Hemostat Angled 90 Deg, FST #13012-12),
    (b) Flat rounded forceps (Standard Pattern Forceps Straight 18 cm, FST # 11000-18),
    (c) Curved pointed forceps with teeth (Graefe Tissue Forceps 10 cm, Roboz #RS-5158),
    (d) Curved pointed forceps (JFA5bTC SuperGrip Forceps Angled 45 Deg, FST #00649-11),
    (e) Curved scissors (Extra Fine Micro Dissecting Scissors, Roboz #RS-5883),

(f) Spring scissors (Vannas Spring Scissors Straight 2 mm Cutting Edge, FST #15000-03).

6. Surgical suture S1 (Mariderm blue (U.S.P. size 5-0), Megro).
7. Surgical suture S2 (Mersilk* (U.S.P. size 5-0), Ethicon).
8. Mouse ear puncher (2 mm punch hole).
9. Povidone-iodine (PVP-I).
10. Hydrating eye gel (Vismed).
11. 0.9% NaCl physiological saline (20 mL and 500 mL).
12. Systemic anesthesia (1 mg/mL of Ketamine (Narketan, Vetoquinol AG), 5 mg/mL of Xylazine (Chanazine, Chanelle Pharmaceuticals), and 0.4 mg/mL of Acepromazine (Promace, Fort Dodge Animal Health).
13. Analgesic (3.5 mg/kg of Ketoprofen (Ketonal, Lek d.d.)).
14. Aminoglycoside antibiotic (Bivacyn, Lek d.d.).
15. 10 mm Petri dishes.
16. Stereo microscope (Stemi 2000-C Stereo Microscope 6.5×–50×, Carl Zeiss).
17. Micropore tape.
18. Ethanol (70%).
19. Depilatory cream (Veet, Reckitt Benckiser).
20. Hair clippers.
21. Weighing scale.
22. 0.5 mL insulin syringe 29 G.
23. Bath container.
24. Heating pad (Rodent Warmer ×1, Stoelting).
25. Retort stand (support stand) with clamped steel rod.
26. Surgical light.
27. Cotton swabs.
28. Round microscope glass slips (diameter 12 mm, thickness 0.16–0.19 mm (APJ trading)).
29. Surgical cotton fabric.
30. 4 mm vertical torque wrench.

2.2 Tumor Induction in the DSWC

1. 80–90% Confluent cell culture of tumor cells producing green fluorescent protein (GFP) reporter (murine breast cancer model 4T1 producing GFP (4T1-GFP)).
2. Growth media: Advanced Roswell Park Memorial Institute (RPMI) 1640 (Gibco™, Thermo Fisher Scientific).
3. Trypsin.
4. Cell counter.

5. 0.5 mL insulin syringe 29 G.
6. Pipette and tips.
7. 0.9% NaCl physiological saline (20 mL).
8. Matrigel Matrix (Matrigel® Basement Membrane Matrix, Phenol Red-free Corning, #356237).
9. Bleu Patente V (25 mg/mL) (Guerbet).
10. Isoflurane (Isoflurin, VetPharma Animal Health).
11. Inhalation anesthesia with induction chamber.
12. Anesthesia cone mask.
13. Povidone-iodine (PVP-I).
14. Cotton swabs.
15. Ice box.
16. Surgical light.

2.3 Splenocyte Isolation and Staining

1. Scissors.
2. Forceps.
3. Glass-cutting board.
4. Two scalpels.
5. Thermoshaker.
6. Cell counter.
7. Fluorescence microscope.
8. Pipette and tips.
9. 10× Red Blood Cell (RBC) Lysis Buffer (BioLegend).
10. Collagenase IV (Worthington Biochemical).
11. Hyaluronidase (Sigma-Aldrich).
12. DNase I (Analytik Jena).
13. Hanks' Balanced Salt Solution (HBSS) buffer (Ca^{2+}, Mg^{2+}) (Gibco™, Thermo Fisher Scientific).
14. Distilled water 500 mL (dH_2O).
15. 1× Phosphate-buffered saline (PBS).
16. 1 mL syringe plunger.
17. 40 μm sterile cell strainer.
18. CellTracker™ CM-DiI Dye (CM-DiI Dye) (Thermo Fisher Scientific).

2.4 Intravenous Splenocyte Injection

1. Polyethylene tube (BTPE-10, 0.28 mm × 0.6 mm, Instech Laboratories).
2. Needles of 0.5 mL insulin syringes 29 G.
3. 0.5 mL insulin syringe 29 G.

4. Isoflurane (Isoflurin, VetPharma Animal Health).
5. Inhalation anesthesia with induction chamber.
6. Anesthesia cone mask.
7. Gauze.
8. Ethanol (70%).
9. Beaker with warm water.
10. Pipette and tips.
11. Suspension of fluorescently labeled splenocytes.
12. Micropore tape.
13. Flat rounded forceps.
14. Surgical light.

2.5 Intravital Imaging of Splenocytes in the DSWC

1. Confocal microscope with motorized stage and Z-stacking (LSM 800, Carl Zeiss).
2. Microscope slide holder.
3. Aluminum DSWC frame holder.
4. 20× water immersion objective (NA 0.8).
5. Ultrasound gel diluted in dH_2O (ratio 2:1).
6. Micropore tape.
7. Adhesive gum.
8. Ethanol (70%).
9. Cotton swabs.
10. Isoflurane (Isoflurin, VetPharma Animal Health).
11. Inhalation anesthesia with induction chamber.
12. Two separate anesthesia tubings with anesthesia cone mask.
13. Heating pad (Rodent Warmer ×1, Stoelting).
14. *Optional:* Lycopersicon Esculentum (Tomato) Lectin (LEL, TL), DyLight™ 649 (LEL-Dye) (1 mg/mL) (Vector Laboratories).

3 Methods

3.1 Implantation of the Dorsal Skinfold Window Chamber (DSWC)

Surgical implantation of the DSWC should be performed using aseptic techniques. Autoclave and sterilize all surgical tools, dorsal window chamber set, gauzes, and surgical cotton fabric before the procedure.

1. All the surgical equipment and the DWSC should be autoclaved before use.
2. Wipe all the surfaces with a disinfectant.

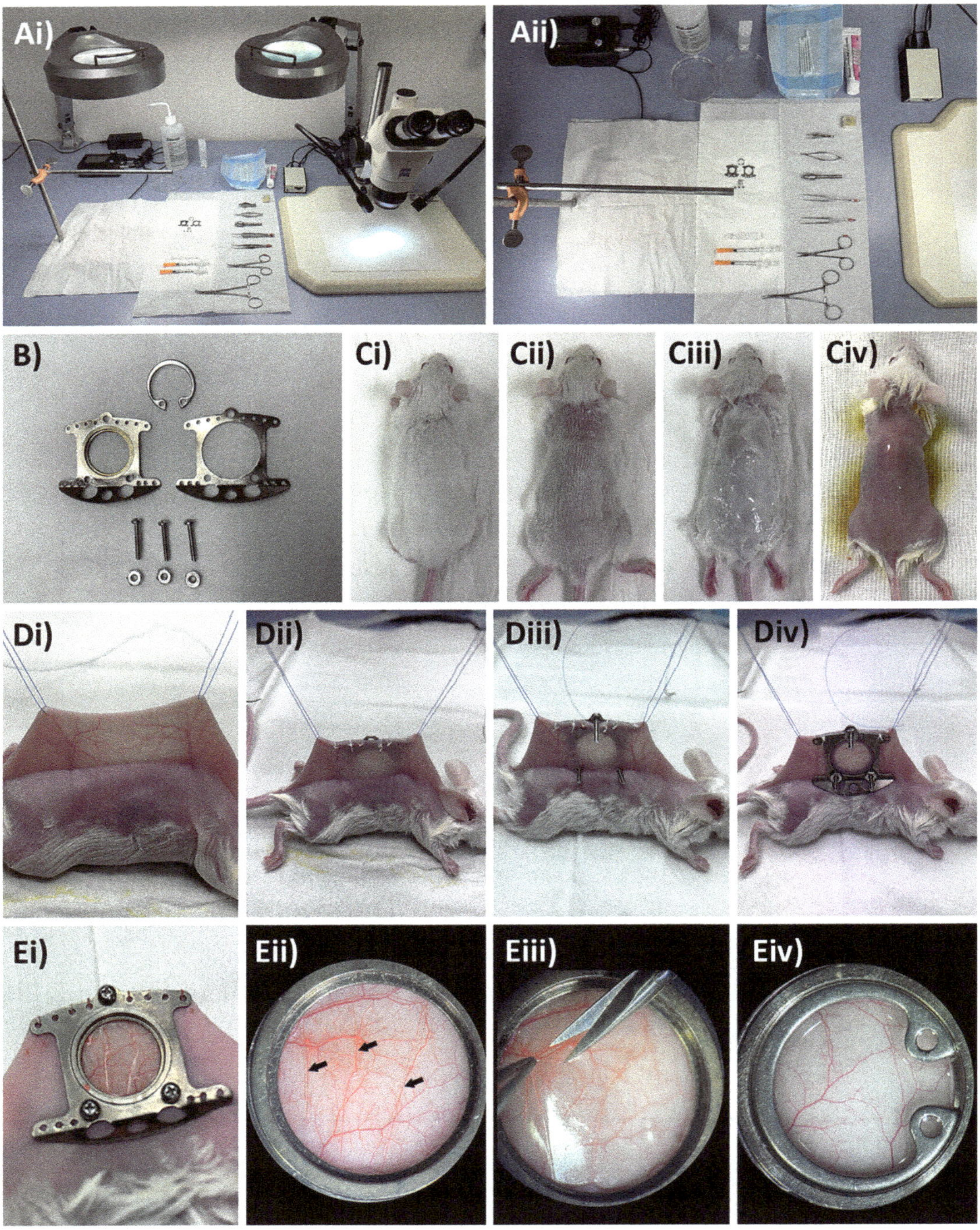

Fig. 1 Implantation of the DSWC. Images show (**Ai**) the operating room, the surgical site, (**Aii**) surgical tools, and (**B**) DSWC components. Images (**Ci**–**Civ**) show the depilation steps. Specifically, (**Ci**) shows the mouse before hair removal, (**Cii**) after hair removal with hair clippers, (**Ciii**) after application of depilatory cream and (**Ciii**) after disinfection of the depilated skin with Povidone-iodine. Images (**Di**–**Div**) show implantation of the DSWC. The skinfold on the back of the mouse is (**Di**) stretched out and suspended with two surgical sutures. (**Dii**) After the first DSWC frame is sewn on, (**Diii**) holes are made through the openings and screws are inserted. (**Div**) The second DSWC frame is attached and tightened with three nuts and four sutures. Images (**Ei**–**Eiv**) show the removal of the upper skin layer and process of closing the DSWC. (**Ei**) The upper skin layer in

3. Prepare the surgical site (Fig. 1Ai, Aii). Place the retort stand on the operating table and place the functioning heating pad on top. Cover the heating pad together with the retort stand and a margin of operating table with sterile surgical cotton fabric. Place another but smaller sterile surgical cotton fabric on top. Provide optimal lighting conditions with a surgical light. Place the microscope near the operating site for easier transfer of mice. Prepare two separate labeled Petri dishes containing 70% ethanol and physiological saline. Place surgical tools on a piece of surgical cotton fabric covering the operating table. Prepare a syringe containing analgesic.
4. Prepare the hair removal site. Prepare a scale, hair clippers, a bath container, separate mouse cage, sterile surgical cotton fabric, and a syringe containing anesthesia.
5. Weigh the mice and administer the appropriate volume of systemic anesthesia by intraperitoneal injection (*see* **Note 1**). Place the mice in the prepared mouse cage.
6. When sedated, place the mouse on the sterile surgical cotton fabric and use hair clippers to remove the hair on the back of the mouse together with a large margin of hair on both lateral sides (Fig. 1Ci, Cii).
7. Apply depilatory cream on the trimmed area for 90 s (Fig. 1Ciii).
8. Soak the gauze in the warm water in a bath container and use it to remove the depilatory cream (*see* **Note 2**).
9. Disinfect the depilated area using Povidone-iodine soaked gauze (Fig. 1Civ).
10. Place the mouse on the working platform underneath the steel rod of the retort stand (*see* **Note 3**), administer 50 μL of analgesic subcutaneously above the neck and apply the hydrating eye gel to prevent corneal drying.
11. Create a skinfold along the back of the mice and align the lateral vessels. Hold the skinfold adjacent to the neck (superior) and pierce near the edge of the skinfold using surgical suture S1. Secure both ends of the surgical suture S1 over the steel rod of the retort stand to suspend and stretch the skinfold. Fix the suture with the Micropore tape. Proceed in the same way at the skinfold adjacent to the tail (inferior) (Fig. 1Di).

Fig. 1 (continued) the DSWC is removed using curved pointed forceps with teeth and curved scissors. (**Eii**) The thin layer of fat has distinct parallel blood vessels marked with black arrows and is (**Eiii**) removed with curved pointed forceps and spring scissors. (**Eiv**) The exposed underlying skin is sealed with microscope glass slip and the clip

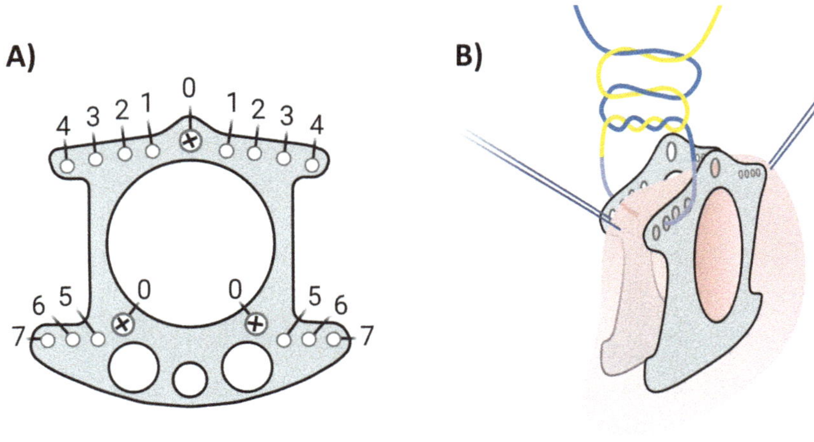

Fig. 2 Mounting of the DSWC. Image (**a**) shows the hole numbers of the DSWC used to sew the first frame to the skinfold, to insert the screws and to sew both frames together. Image (**b**) shows surgeon's throw followed by two additional alternating throws. For a secure knot, however, it is recommended to perform four additional alternating throws

12. Position the first dorsal window chamber frame behind the suspended skinfold and use surgical suture S2 to stitch the frame to the edge of the skinfold through the holes numbered 1, 2, and 4 (Figs. 1Dii and 2a). Loosely tighten each suture with a secure knot consisting of surgeon's throw followed by four additional alternating throws (Fig. 2b) (*see* **Note 4**).
13. Punch two holes on the bottom part of the skinfold with the mouse ear puncher and insert the screws (Fig. 1Diii). Align the other dorsal window chamber frame to fit through the screws (Fig. 1Div).
14. Place the nuts on all three screws and loosely tighten them using the vertical torque wrench. Remove the sutures S2. Sew the frames and the skinfold in between together with a surgical suture S2 through the holes numbered 3, 5, and 6 (Fig. 2a).
15. Place the mouse on its side with the window hole facing upward. Carefully cut out the upper layer of the skin using curved pointed forceps with teeth and curved scissors (Fig. 1Ei) (*see* **Note 5**).
16. Transfer the working platform together with the mouse under the stereo microscope and examine the exposed underlying skin in the dorsal window chamber.
17. Remove the thin layer of fat using curved pointed forceps and spring scissors under the stereo microscope (Fig. 1Eii, Eiii) (*see* **Note 6**).
18. If necessary, gently wash the exposed underlying skin with physiological saline and sterilized cotton swabs.

19. Apply physiological saline to the exposed underlying skin and place the microscope glass slip on top without introducing any air bubbles. Using pean forceps seal the window chamber with the clip (Fig. 1Eiv).
20. Apply the antibiotic around the stitches with cotton swabs and place the mouse in an empty, clean cage (*see* **Note 7**).
21. Place the cage on a separate heating pad and reapply the eye hydrating gel if needed. Observe the mouse for 1 h until the anesthesia wears off.

3.2 Tumor Induction in the DSWC

Tumor induction should be performed 24 h after the implantation of the DSWC to avoid prolonging the duration of the procedure and to minimize animal discomfort. For tumor induction, prepare in advance 80–90% confluent cell culture containing at least 10×10^6 of tumor cells producing GFP reporter (4T1-GFP). One day before the tumor induction thaw the Matrigel Matrix on 4 °C. While preparing the cell suspension, keep the cells on ice. Use cooled pipette tips when pipetting the Matrigel Matrix to avoid its polymerization.

1. Prepare the cell suspension by aspirating the media from the cell culture flask. Wash the cells with 10 mL of 1× PBS. Add 3 mL of trypsin and aspirate after 30 s. Incubate the cells in the flask for 1 min in the incubator. Add 10 mL of growth media (Advanced RPMI-1640) and transfer the cell suspension to a 50 mL centrifuge tube. Centrifuge the cells at 300 × *g* for 5 min. Aspirate the growth media and add 1 mL of physiological saline. Count the cells using cell counter while keeping the cell suspension on ice.
2. Transfer the 5×10^6 of cells to a new 50 mL centrifuge tube. Centrifuge the cells at 300 × *g* for 5 min at 4 °C. Aspirate the physiological saline. Add 50 μL of physiological saline to the pellet and resuspend. Using cooled pipette tips add 45 μL of Matrigel Matrix and 5 μL of Bleu Patente V to the cell suspension (*see* **Note 8**).
3. Prepare an ice box containing the cell suspension, pipette tips and a syringe (*see* **Note 9**).
4. Anesthetize the mouse in the anesthesia induction chamber under 2% (v/v) of isoflurane.
5. When anesthetized, fit the mouse muzzle to the anesthesia cone mask.
6. Place the mouse on its side to expose the skin opposite to the cover slip in the dorsal window chamber and examine the target area (Fig. 3a) (*see* **Note 10**).
7. Disinfect the area using Povidone-iodine and cotton swabs.

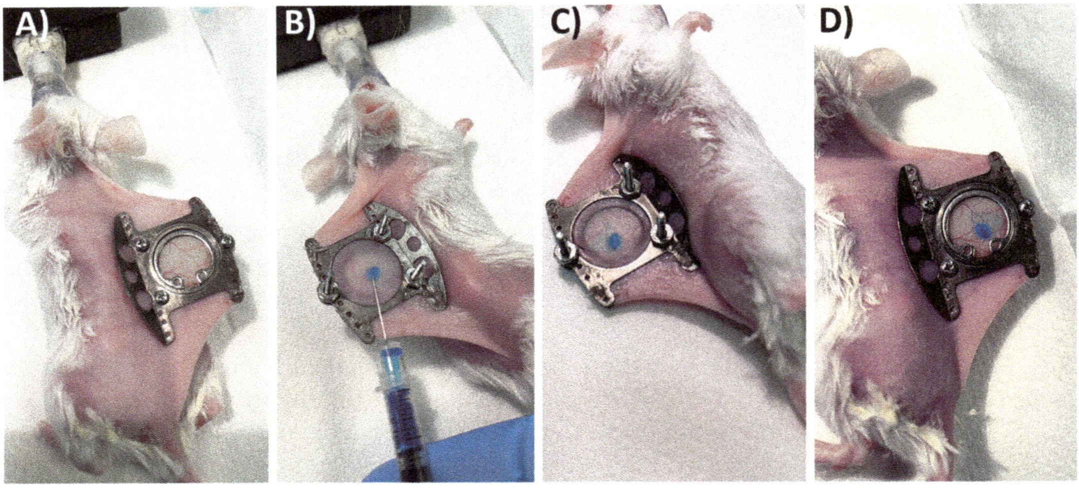

Fig. 3 Tumor induction in the DSWC. (**a**) The DSWC of a mouse under inhalation is first inspected, and the target area for tumor induction is determined. (**b**) The needle of a syringe containing tumor cells producing GFP reporter, mixed with Matrigel Matrix and Bleu Patente V, is inserted underneath the skin and (**c**) tumor cell suspension is injected. (**d**) Successful tumor induction is indicated by a blue bulge

8. Load the syringe with 100 μL of the prepared cell suspension (*see* **Note 11**). Place the tip of the loaded insulin syringe parallel to the skin near the window frame. Under minimal angle pierce the skin and continue toward the middle. Carefully inject 5 μL of cell suspension (containing 2.5×10^6 tumor cells producing GFP reporter) and wait for 5 s before completely exiting the injection site (Fig. 3b–d).
9. Return the mouse in the cage and observe in the upcoming days. Tumors should reach a volume of 25 mm^3 (calculated using formula: $V = a \times b^2 \times \pi/6$) on day 10.

3.3 Splenocyte Isolation and Staining

Naive splenocytes are isolated from the spleen of a healthy donor mouse. Approximately 100 million splenocytes can be isolated from a single donor spleen. When taking into the account the losses during staining and the dead volume of the syringe for intravenous injection in mice, the number of labeled splenocytes may be sufficient for 10 applications.

Prior to splenocyte isolation and staining, dilute the 10× RBC Lysis Buffer in deionized water to 1× working concentration. Prepare the mixture of collagenase IV (3.2 mg/mL) and hyaluronidase (0.32 mg/mL) in 5 mL of HBSS (Ca^{2+}, Mg^{2+}) with 2 U/mL of DNase I.

1. Euthanize the donor mouse by cervical dislocation.
2. Using scissors and forceps cut the left lateral side of the mouse, excise and transfer the spleen on a clean glass cutting board (*see* **Note 12**).

3. Add 200 μL of the collagenase and hyaluronidase mixture to the spleen and homogenize it mechanically using two scalpels (*see* **Note 13**).
4. Transfer the homogenized spleen to a 50 mL centrifuge tube containing 5 mL of collagenase and hyaluronidase mixture. Place the suspension on ice.
5. Incubate the suspension for 30 min with shaking (150 rpm) at 37 °C (*see* **Note 14**).
6. Transfer the suspension through a 40 μm sterile cell strainer.
7. Using a 1 mL pipette and a syringe plunger, wash the cell strainer with 5 mL of 1× PBS (*see* **Note 15**).
8. Centrifuge the filtrate for 5 min at 400 × *g* and 4 °C. Discard the supernatant.
9. Wash the pellet with 2 mL of 1× PBS and repeat the centrifugation step. Discard the supernatant.
10. Resuspend the pellet in 5 mL of 1× RBC Lysis Buffer.
11. Incubate on ice for 5 min with occasional shaking.
12. Stop the reaction by diluting 1× RBC Lysis Buffer with 20 mL of 1× PBS.
13. Centrifuge (5 min, 400 × *g*, 4 °C) and discard the supernatant.
14. Resuspend splenocytes in 1 mL of HBSS (Ca^{2+}, Mg^{2+}) and count.
15. Dilute 50 μL of stock (1000 μM) CM-DiI Dye solution in 10 mL of HBSS (Ca^{2+}, Mg^{2+}) to a final concentration of 5 μM.
16. Resuspend 10×10^6 splenocytes in 1 mL HBSS (Ca^{2+}, Mg^{2+}) containing CM-DiI Dye. Prepare 10 samples in separate 1.5 mL microcentrifuge tubes.
17. Incubate the splenocyte suspension for 15 min with shaking (400 rpm) at 37 °C, followed by 15 min incubation on ice (*see* **Note 16**).
18. Combine the splenocyte suspension of all 10 samples in a 50 mL centrifuge tube and centrifuge (400 × *g*, 5 min, 4 °C). Discard the supernatant, wash with 1 mL of 1× PBS and centrifuge again.
19. Resuspend labeled splenocytes in 1 mL of physiological saline (*see* **Note 17**). Keep the cells on ice.
20. Count labeled splenocytes using cell counter and calculate the volume needed to prepare 50×10^6 splenocytes per mL.
21. Transfer the required volume of labeled splenocytes in a new 1.5 mL microcentrifuge tube and add physiological saline to a final volume of 1 mL.

22. Keep the labeled splenocyte suspension on ice and resuspend before use.

3.4 Intravenous Splenocyte Injection

Intravenous injection of fluorescently labeled splenocytes in mice should be performed immediately after splenocyte isolation and staining. Before the procedure, use flat rounded forceps to break off the needle tips of insulin syringes. Cut the polyethylene tubing into 15 cm and 10 cm long pieces. Insert broken end of a needle tip on one end of each polyethylene tubes. On the other end of 15 cm polyethylene tube, attach a syringe containing physiological saline (*see* **Note 18**). On the other end of 10 cm polyethylene tube, attach a syringe containing splenocyte suspension. The syringe containing splenocyte suspension should be kept on ice before application.

1. Anesthetize the mouse in the anesthesia induction chamber under 2% (v/v) of isoflurane.
2. When anesthetized, fit the mouse muzzle to the anesthesia cone mask. Apply eye drops to the eyes to prevent corneal drying.
3. Place the mouse on its side to expose one of the lateral tail veins.
4. Submerge the tail in the beaker containing warm water (30–37 °C) for 30 s (Fig. 4a) (*see* **Note 19**).
5. Dry the tail with fresh gauze. Sterilize the tail with gauze soaked in 70% ethanol.
6. Place the tip of a needle attached to the polyethylene tube and syringe containing physiological saline parallel to the skin above the lateral vein and pierce it under minimal angle (*see* **Note 20**). Penetration of the vein can be recognized by the pressure drop. Carefully continue along the vein and insert half of the needle (Fig. 4b).
7. To verify that the needle is inside the vein slowly inject physiological saline. Correct insertion of the needle is identified by no resistance and no formation of the bulge (Fig. 4c).
8. Once the needle is inserted use the Micropore tape to fix the polyethylene tube together with the tail (Fig. 4d).
9. Cut off the polyethylene tube near the insertion site. Connect the tip of the needle attached to the polyethylene tube and the syringe containing the splenocyte suspension.
10. Slowly inject 100 μL of splenocyte suspension (containing 5×10^6 labeled splenocytes) (Fig. 4e).
11. Carefully remove the tip of the needle attached to the polyethylene tube and syringe containing splenocyte suspension, which can be reused.

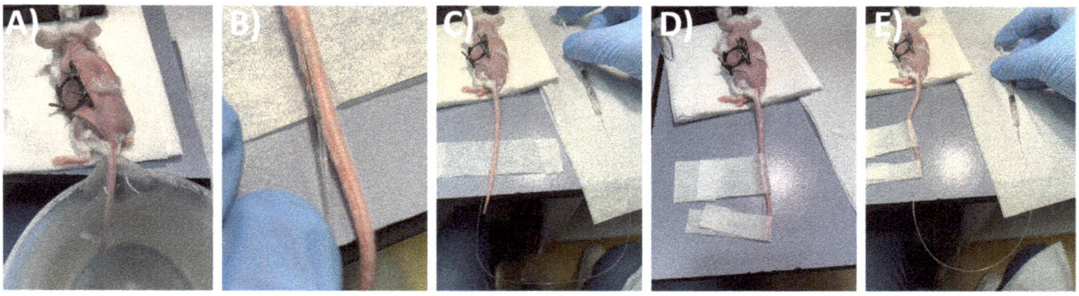

Fig. 4 Intravenous splenocyte application. (**a**) To induce vasodilatation the tail is first submerged in warm water. (**b**) The tip of a needle attached to the polyethylene tube and a syringe containing physiological saline is inserted into the lateral vein of the tail. (**c**) Physiological saline is injected to verify that the needle is inside the vein. (**d**) Micropore tape is used to fix the polyethylene tube together with the tail and the polyethylene tube is cut off. (**e**) The needle attached to the polyethylene tube and the syringe containing splenocyte suspension is connected to the cut-off polyethylene tube, and the splenocyte suspension is slowly injected

12. Remove the micropore tape and the tip of the needle attached to the cut-off polyethylene tube from the vein.

3.5 Intravital Imaging of Splenocytes in the DSWC

Extravasation of splenocytes into tumors is a spatiotemporal event. Therefore, intravital imaging of fluorescently labeled splenocytes and their migration into tumors in the DSWC is performed at multiple time points (typically 4, 24, and 48 h) after intravenous application.

1. Prepare the imaging site. Clear and sterilize the imaging table and the stage of the confocal microscope. Insert the microscope slide holder into the stage opening and position the two sliders of the microscope slide holder to fit the aluminum DSWC frame holder. Prepare the inhalation anesthesia with the induction chamber and two separate anesthesia tubings with anesthesia cone masks. The anesthesia tubing with the anesthesia cone mask placed on the table is used to prepare the DSWC, while the other is fixed on top of the motorized stage to reduce animals' movement during intravital imaging (*see* **Note 21**). To maintain normal body temperature of the mouse during imaging, fix the heating pad on the stage and turn it on before imaging.
2. Anesthetize the mouse in the anesthesia induction chamber under 2% (v/v) of isoflurane.
3. When anesthetized, fit the mouse muzzle to the anesthesia cone mask of the anesthesia tubing placed on the table. Apply eye drops to the eyes to prevent corneal drying (*see* **Note 22**).
4. Examine the DSWC and tighten any loose nuts using the vertical torque wrench. Place the mouse on the side and clean the microscope glass slip of the DSWC with cotton swabs dipped in 70% ethanol.

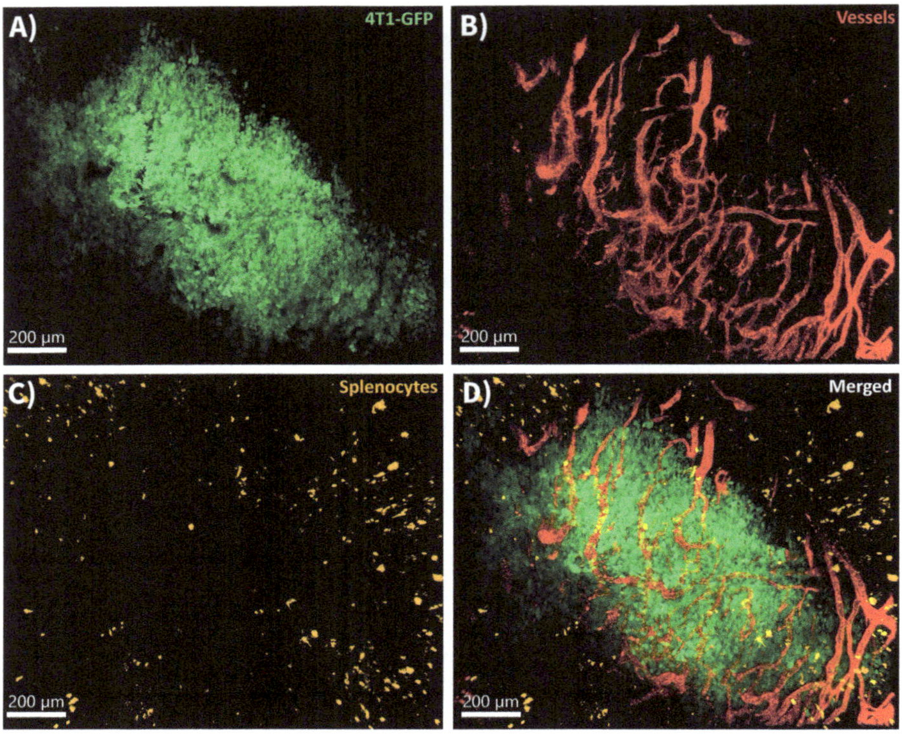

Fig. 5 Intravital imaging of splenocytes in the DSWC. Images (**a**–**d**) show stitched and stacked images after intravital imaging of the DSWC processed with Imaris software (Bitplane). Images (**a**–**d**) represent individual channels, where (**a**) represents 4T1 tumor cells producing GFP reporter (green, GFP), (**b**) vessels (red, LEL-Dye), (**c**) splenocytes (yellow, CM-Dil Dye), and (**d**) merged image. Scale bar: 200 µm

5. Fit the screws of the DSWC through the openings on the aluminum DSWC frame holder and tighten three nuts on the backside of the frame using the vertical torque wrench.
6. Transfer the mouse onto the stage of the confocal microscope and fit the mouse muzzle to the anesthesia cone mask of the anesthesia tubing placed on the table. Place the mouse on its side so that the microscope glass slip of the DSWC is positioned upward. Fit the aluminum DSWC frame holder between the two preset sliders of the microscope slide holder. To further prevent animals' movement and interference with the objective during image acquisition, secure the lower part of the mouse and the tail with a Micropore tape onto the stage.
7. Apply diluted ultrasound gel between the 20× immersion objective and the microscope glass slip of the DSWC. Manually position the DSWC in the center and slowly lower the objective.
8. First, manually focus the image through the oculars and locate the GFP positive tumor cells by using the laser with excitation wavelength of 488 nm and setting the variable dichroic and

filters at channel specific wavelength between 488 and 545 nm (GFP). Determine the total region of interest.

9. Enter the acquisition mode. Set the appropriate acquisition speed, resolution, and image size. Activate the lasers with excitation wavelengths of 488 nm and 561 nm and set the variable dichroic and filters at channel specific wavelength: 488–545 nm (GFP) and 565–620 nm (CM-DiI Dye) (*see* **Note 23**). To capture only the fluorescence emission peak, use appropriate short-pass and long-pass filters.
10. Enable the Tiles option. Set the number of tiles to capture the entire region of interest.
11. Enable the Z-stacking option. Set the first and the last image plane along the Z-axis with 5 μm spacing between individual image planes.
12. Enable channel voltage interpolation and set the appropriate channel voltage used to capture the first, center, and the last image plane along the *Z* axis.
13. Start the image acquisition. Depending on the number of tiles and the imaging depth, the image acquisition can take up to 45 min per mouse. Monitor the mouse breathing and reduce the percentage of isoflurane anesthesia, if needed, during image acquisition.
14. After imaging the last time point, euthanize the mouse immediately after the image acquisition.
15. After imaging, preprocess the .czi image files by fusing individual captured tiles into a seamless image by applying the Stitching method.
16. Export and analyze images using adequate image processing software such as Imaris (Bitplane) (Fig. 5a–d).

4 Notes

1. Recommended volumes for administered anesthesia based on mouse weight and mouse line are gathered in Table 1.
2. Remove all of the depilatory cream, otherwise the skin will become irritated and inoperable due to inflammation. Repeat the process and reapply the depilatory cream where the hair remains. Unremoved hair can overgrow the region of interest and interfere during image acquisition.
3. The orientation of the mouse determines the placement of the window chamber. If the mouse is facing to your right-hand side than the frame containing the window will be located on the left lateral side of the mouse and vice versa.

Table 1
Recommended volumes for administered anesthesia

Weight (g)/Mouse line	C57Bl/6 V (μL)	BALB/c V (μL)
<17.5	Too low	Too low
17.5–18	90	100
18–18.5	100	100
18.5–19.5	105	105
19.6–20.5	120	110
20.6–21.5	125	120
21.6–22.5	125	125

Mice weighing below 17.5 g should be excluded from the experiment

4. The first throw, however, should be loosely tightened to prevent the constriction of the blood flow.
5. Cut all the skin around the edges of the window to prevent skin regrowth.
6. The thin layer of fat can be distinguished by characteristic parallel blood vessels. Removing the layer of fat will reduce the rate of healing process, macrophage infiltration and result in clearer images. This step should be done with extreme caution as interruption of blood vessels and blood accumulation often leads to inflammation.
7. Place the mouse on a surgical cotton fabric but do not introduce any environmental enrichments, food cradle or other objects, which could cause the entanglement of the dorsal window chamber frame.
8. Matrigel Matrix is composed of four major basement membrane ECM proteins: laminin (~60%), collagen IV (~30%), entactin (~8%), and the heparin sulfate proteoglycan perlecan (~2–3%) which facilitate tumor growth. Bleu Patente V is a synthetic dye used for various perioperative indications and in the case of tumor induction helps to visualize the extent and distribution of the injected cell suspension.
9. Before tumor induction, all mice and the DSWCs should be inspected and any inflammation or tissue damage should be attended before proceeding. Stitches, screws and nuts should be examined and tightened if needed. If the DSWC is inflamed or containing a blood clot, remove the clip together with the microscope glass slip and clean the exposed area with a sterile cotton swab. After cleaning, apply the physiological saline and seal the window with a new microscope glass slip and the clip.

10. The target area for injecting the tumor cell suspension should be determined based on the location of vessels, but preferably in the middle of the window chamber. If vessels are in the way tumor cell suspension is preferably injected in the upper area of the window chamber. It is common that the skin in the dorsal window chamber loosens up before imaging, causing tumors in the upper part to relocate to the middle.
11. Before loading the syringe, resuspend the cell suspension with cooled pipette tips.
12. Clean the glass cutting board with dH_2O and 70% ethanol using gauze. Let the glass cutting board air-dry for 1 min.
13. Mechanical homogenization increases the surface of the reactant and thereby speeds up enzymatic degradation of connective tissue by increasing collagenase and hyaluronidase reaction rate.
14. To reduce the overall time of the procedure set the thermoshaker to 37 °C before start. Place the 50 mL centrifuge in the thermoshaker at 60-degree angle for a better enzyme distribution.
15. Wash the cell strainer filter in steps. First wash the cell strainer with 1 mL of 1× PBS, then use the syringe plunger and gently press along the cell strainer membrane. Repeat 4 times to maximize the isolation efficiency.
16. Aliquoting isolated splenocytes into 10 smaller fractions and longer incubation times improve their labeling.
17. Verify that the labeling was successful by transferring 10 μL of the splenocyte suspension on the objective slide and examine under a fluorescence microscope.
18. Needle tip attached to the polyethylene tube and a syringe allows for more precise manipulation and administration. Needle tip attached to the 15 cm polyethylene tube and the syringe containing physiological saline allows for multiple applications and serves as an indicator of successful intravenous insertion. With each application the tube is cut off near the needle tip and gets shorter (*see* **step 9**).
19. Incubation of the tail in warm water will cause vasodilatation and easier insertion of the needle into the vein. Optionally, exposure of the tail to the infrared light can be used to achieve the same effect.
20. To inspect the area of injection run the needle tip through the skin and the underlying vein.

    This step will ensure that the needle will stay inside the vein during the procedure.

21. To fix the anesthesia tubing with anesthesia cone mask on the stage use adhesive gum and Micropore tape. Ensure that the anesthesia tubing does not interfere with the movement of the motorized stage.
22. *Optional:* To fluorescently label the vessels perform intravenous administration of LEL-Dye by following the same steps as for the administration of splenocytes in Subheading 3.4. Administer 70 μL (1 mg/mL) of the dye 1 h prior to imaging.
23. *Optional:* To capture vessels labeled with (LEL-Dye) activate laser with excitation wavelength of 640 nm and set the variable dichroic and filters at channel specific wavelength between 645 and 700 nm (LEL-Dye).

Acknowledgments

This work was supported by research program P3-0003.

References

1. Galluzzi L, Chan TA, Kroemer G et al (2018) The hallmarks of successful anticancer immunotherapy. Sci Transl Med 10:1–15. https://doi.org/10.1126/scitranslmed.aat7807
2. Gao G, Wang Z, Qu X, Zhang Z (2020) Prognostic value of tumor-infiltrating lymphocytes in patients with triple-negative breast cancer: a systematic review and meta-analysis. BMC Cancer 20:179. https://doi.org/10.1186/s12885-020-6668-z
3. Zhang Y, Zhang Z (2020) The history and advances in cancer immunotherapy: understanding the characteristics of tumor-infiltrating immune cells and their therapeutic implications. Cell Mol Immunol 17:807–821. https://doi.org/10.1038/s41423-020-0488-6
4. Blair TC, Alice AF, Zebertavage L et al (2021) The dynamic entropy of tumor immune infiltrates: the impact of recirculation, antigen-specific interactions, and retention on T cells in tumors. Front Oncol 11:1–21. https://doi.org/10.3389/fonc.2021.653625
5. Okla K, Farber DL, Zou W (2021) Tissue-resident memory T cells in tumor immunity and immunotherapy. J Exp Med 218:1–14. https://doi.org/10.1084/jem.20201605
6. Li T, Fu J, Zeng Z et al (2020) TIMER2.0 for analysis of tumor-infiltrating immune cells. Nucleic Acids Res 48:W509–W514. https://doi.org/10.1093/NAR/GKAA407
7. Li B, Severson E, Pignon JC et al (2016) Comprehensive analyses of tumor immunity: implications for cancer immunotherapy. Genome Biol 17:1–16. https://doi.org/10.1186/s13059-016-1028-7
8. Shelton SE, Nguyen HT, Barbie DA, Kamm RD (2021) Engineering approaches for studying immune-tumor cell interactions and immunotherapy. iScience 24:101985. https://doi.org/10.1016/j.isci.2020.101985
9. Fomitcheva-Khartchenko A, Kashyap A, Geiger T, Kaigala GV (2022) Space in cancer biology: its role and implications. Trends Cancer 8:1019–1032. https://doi.org/10.1016/j.trecan.2022.07.008
10. Lian N, Oren R, Filip B, Michal N (2014) Imaging aspects of the tumor stroma with therapeutic implications. Pharmacol Ther 141:192–208. https://doi.org/10.1016/j.pharmthera.2013.10.003
11. Li C, Shan S, Braun RD, Dewhirst MW (2000) Initial stages of tumor cell-induced angiogenesis: evaluation via skin window chambers in rodent models. J Natl Cancer Inst 92:143–147
12. Biel NM, Lee JA, Sorg BS, Siemann DW (2014) Limitations of the dorsal skinfold window chamber model in evaluating anti-angiogenic therapy during early phase of angiogenesis. Vasc Cell 6:1–11. https://doi.org/10.1186/2045-824X-6-17
13. Kaskas NM, Moore-Medlin T, McClure GB et al (2014) Serum biomarkers in head and

neck squamous cell cancer. JAMA Otolaryngol Head Neck Surg 140:5–11. https://doi.org/10.1001/jamaoto.2013.5688

14. Markelc B, Bellard E, Sersa G et al (2018) Increased permeability of blood vessels after reversible electroporation is facilitated by alterations in endothelial cell-to-cell junctions. J Control Release 276:30–41. https://doi.org/10.1016/j.jconrel.2018.02.032
15. Markelc B, Sersa G, Cemazar M (2013) Differential mechanisms associated with vascular disrupting action of electrochemotherapy: intravital microscopy on the level of single normal and tumor blood vessels. PLoS One 8:1–11. https://doi.org/10.1371/journal.pone.0059557
16. Hak S, Reitan NK, Haraldseth O, De Lange DC (2010) Intravital microscopy in window chambers: a unique tool to study tumor angiogenesis and delivery of nanoparticles. Angiogenesis 13:113–130. https://doi.org/10.1007/s10456-010-9176-y
17. Perrone F, Craparo EF, Cemazar M et al (2021) Targeted delivery of siRNAs against hepatocellular carcinoma-related genes by a galactosylated polyaspartamide copolymer. J Control Release 330:1132–1151. https://doi.org/10.1016/j.jconrel.2020.11.020
18. Murty S, Haile ST, Beinat C et al (2020) Intravital imaging reveals synergistic effect of CAR T-cells and radiation therapy in a preclinical immunocompetent glioblastoma model. Onco Targets Ther 9. https://doi.org/10.1080/2162402X.2020.1757360
19. Savarin M, Prevc A, Rzek M et al (2018) Intravital monitoring of vasculature after targeted gene therapy alone or combined with tumor irradiation. Technol Cancer Res Treat 17:1–8. https://doi.org/10.1177/1533033818784208
20. Zhang M, Chakraborty SK, Sampath P et al (2015) Fluoromodule-based reporter/probes designed for in vivo fluorescence imaging. J Clin Invest 125:3915–3927. https://doi.org/10.1172/JCI81086
21. Hong S, Pawel GT, Pei R, Lu Y (2021) Recent progress in developing fluorescent probes for imaging cell metabolites. Biomed Mater 16:044108. https://doi.org/10.1088/1748-605X/abfd11
22. Seynhaeve ALB, Ten Hagen TLM (2018) Intravital microscopy of tumor-associated vasculature using advanced dorsal skinfold window chambers on transgenic fluorescent mice. J Vis Exp 2018:1–10. https://doi.org/10.3791/55115
23. Ng TSC, Allen HH, Rashidian M, Miller MA (2022) Probing immune infiltration dynamics in cancer by in vivo imaging. Curr Opin Chem Biol 67:102117. https://doi.org/10.1016/j.cbpa.2022.102117

Chapter 14

Mouse Melanoma Model in Tumor Vaccines and Immunotherapy Research

Mariangela De Robertis, Urša Lampreht Tratar, Emanuela Signori, Tilen Komel, and Maja Čemažar

Abstract

Efficacy of novel cancer immunization protocols could be tested in cell line-derived xenograft tumor models (CDX), which are based on the implantation of human tumor cell lines into mice for the development of different tumors by numerous means, such as subcutaneous implantation and orthotopic, venial, or peritoneal injections. However, the disadvantages of this model are the biological alteration of the derived cells or the inability of the cell lines to accurately reflect the complexity of tumor heterogeneity. Therefore, syngeneic mouse models, which offer a relatively simple grafting technique, preservation of lineage hierarchy, and the ability to generate tumors in as little as 2–8 weeks, are being used to study potential future applications in medical treatment, particularly immunotherapies. Here, we describe a B16.F10 C57Bl/6 mouse melanoma model we selected for therapeutic studies employing IL-2 and IL-12 immunization protocols. Procedure of tumor cells inoculation and melanoma development in mice is described in detail, as first and necessary set-up for successful immunization experiments.

Key words Xenograft mouse models, Cancer immunization, Mouse melanoma model

1 Introduction

Cell line-derived xenograft tumor models (CDX) are frequently used tumor mouse models for the evaluation of in vivo efficacy of novel cancer vaccination strategies. These models are well established with a long history of tumor model characterization, for the assessment of multiple factors involved in the development of malignancies, metastasis, and their response to different types of treatments [1]. CDX are based on the implantation of human tumor cell lines into mice to establish tumor models by numerous means, including subcutaneous implantation and orthotopic, venial, or peritoneal injection [1].

During generation of cancer cell lines, a limitation could be the possible alteration of the biological properties of the derived cells.

Maja Čemažar, Tanja Jesenko and Urša Lampreht Tratar (eds.), *Mouse Models of Cancer: Methods and Protocols*, Methods in Molecular Biology, vol. 2773, https://doi.org/10.1007/978-1-0716-3714-2_14,
© The Author(s), under exclusive license to Springer Science+Business Media, LLC, part of Springer Nature 2024

In this case, CDX could have limited predictive value for cancer therapy. Another disadvantage of this model is linked to the inability of cell lines to not accurately reflect the complexity of tumor heterogeneity, specifically immune component of the tumor microenvironment [2]. Therefore, the use of mouse tumor cell lines growing in immunocompetent mice could represent an advantage for evaluation of vaccination and immune therapies, due to its relative simplicity of the grafting technique. In addition, mouse tumor models allow to generate tumors in only 2–8 weeks [3].

In addition, the use of immunocompromised mice can avoid graft versus host reaction of the mouse against the human tumor tissue, as in the case also of patient-derived xenografts (PDXs) tumor models, which can be generated by implanting surgically removed tumor fragments from patients into immunocompromised animals [4]. However, their deficient immune systems make CDX and PDX models unsuitable for evaluating cancer vaccination strategies. To overcome this limitation, humanized PDX models have recently been implemented with an immune system that is autologous to the implanted tumor [5] or with a human immune system [6], making it possible to use them as models for immunotherapy studies. On the other hand, mouse tumor models in immunocompetent mice can represent a first step in cancer vaccines and cancer immune therapy studies, due to its availability, low cost, and relative simplicity in terms of engrafting.

Tumor cell lines are characterized by different latency periods (generally 10–20 days) before a tumor starts to grow. An important step to consider when setting up an experimental protocol is to establish the right number of cells to be inoculated. A titration curve made by different numbers of cells could be crucial for the success of the experiment. A correct number of cells to consider depends on the parameters crucial for the study, such as site and modality of inoculation, different time scales for tumor development, tumor growth rate curve, tumor microenvironment, maximum tumor mass volume allowed by bioethical criteria with respect to the defined experimental timetable, etc.

Mouse tumor models have been successfully used for the evaluation of cancer vaccines and cytokines immunotherapy. For example, a B16.F10 C57Bl/6 mouse melanoma model was selected for therapeutic studies with IL-2 and IL-12 immunization protocols [7–9]. Here below, we describe the procedure of tumor cell inoculation and melanoma development in mice as first set-up for successful immunization experiments, and the use of LPS (Lipopolysaccharide) injection as a positive control [8, 9] for infiltration of immune cells detected by hematoxylin eosin (H&E) and immunohistochemistry.

2 Materials

- B16.F10 murine melanoma cell line.
- Advanced minimum essential medium (AMEM).
- 5% fetal bovine serum (FBS).
- 10 mL/L L-glutamine.
- 100 U/mL penicillin.
- 50 μg/mL gentamicin.
- 5% CO_2 humidified incubator at 37 °C.
- Trypsin EDTA.
- 6–8-week-old female C57Bl/6 mice weighing 19–23 g.
- Vernier caliper.
- Lipopolysaccharide (LPS).
- Antibodies:
  - Macrophages (*see* **Note 1**).
  - Dendritic cells (*see* **Note 2**).
  - Secondary antibodies (*see* **Note 3**).
- HRP-conjugated avidin staining kit (*see* **Note 4**).
- 10 mM Sodium citrate buffer (pH = 6).
- 3,30-diaminobenzidine (DAB).
- Photomicroscope (*see* **Note 5**).

3 Methods

3.1 Cell Preparation

1. Thaw the tumor cell line and culture the B16.F10 murine melanoma cell line in AMEM supplemented with 5% FBS, 10 mL/L L-glutamine, 100 U/mL penicillin, and 50 μg/mL gentamicin in a 5% CO_2 humidified incubator at 37 °C.
2. When cells reach a confluency of approximately 80%, trypsinize the cells according to the manufacturer instructions.
3. After the trypsinization, inactivate the trypsins with the same amount of cell culture media containing 10% FBS.
4. Collect the cell suspension and centrifuge for 5 min at 300 × *g*.
5. Remove the supernatant and wash the pellet with 5 mL of physiological saline and centrifuge again for 5 min at 300 × *g*.
6. Then resuspend the pellet in appropriate volume of sterile physiological saline (depending on the number of cells required) and count the cells.

7. Prepare 3×10^5 B16.F10 murine melanoma cells resuspended in 100 μL sterile saline solution.

3.2 Tumor Induction by Cell Injection

1. Place the mouse (C57Bl/6) under anesthesia using isoflurane and display right flank of the mouse (that was previously shaven; *see* **Note 6**).
2. Disinfect the injection site of the skin with the disinfectant.
3. By slightly raising the skin fold of the injection site, insert the needle (G29) in the subcutaneous region and inject the cell suspension (*see* **Notes 7** and **8**).

3.3 Tumor Growth Measurements and Animal Survival Curve

1. Observe the mice twice a week for initial tumor development and growth.
2. Additionally monitor the animal's body weight and the general condition of the animal twice a week.
3. After the establishment of the tumor, measure the tumor three times per week using Vernier calipers.
4. Calculate the tumor volumes using the following equation: $V = a \times b \times c \times \pi/6$, where a, b, and c represent the perpendicular diameters of the tumor.
5. Using the data from tumor measurement, draw an animal survival curve (Fig. 1).
6. When the tumors reach 350 mm^3, euthanize the animal.

3.4 Infiltration of LPS as a Positive Control for the Infiltration of Immune Cells

1. Prepare the LPS solution (concentration of 2 mg/mL in physiological saline).
2. When tumors reach 50 mm^3, inject 25 μL LPS (2 mg/mL; 50 μg in total) into the tumor.
3. Harvest the tumors on day 3 or day 7 after LPS injection when the peak of immune cell infiltration is expected.
4. Place the tumors in the formalin free zinc fixative for 24 h and then transferred to 70% ethanol.
5. Embed the fixated tissue into the paraffin blocks.

3.5 Immunohistochemistry Staining

1. Cut the paraffin block into 2 μm thick section for H&E staining according to standard procedures.
2. Cut the paraffin block into 4 μm sections for the immunohistochemistry staining.
3. Carry out the immunohistochemistry by using different primary antibodies to detect the presence of macrophages and dendritic cells (*see* **Note 9**).
4. Before the use of the CD11c antibody, carry out the antigen retrieval procedure in sodium citrate buffer (10 mM sodium

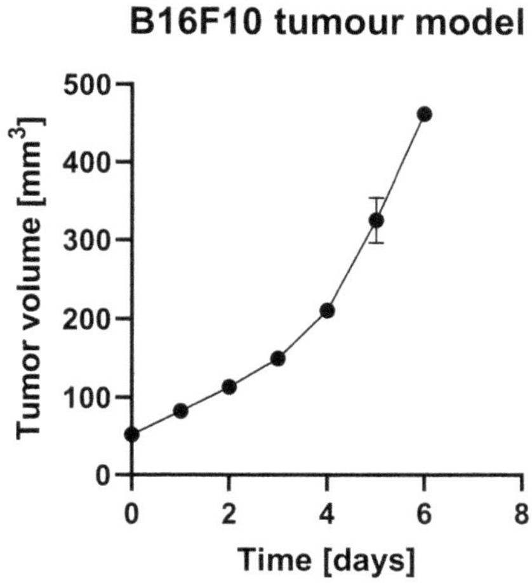

Fig. 1 Growth curve of B16F10 tumors in C57Bl/6 mice

citrate, pH = 6) for 60 min at 95 °C. No retrieval methods needed for the other antibodies.

5. Incubate in a humid chamber overnight at 4 °C with the following primary antibodies (used at a 1:100 dilution in blocking buffer): rat anti-mouse F4/80 clone BM8, rat anti-mouse MHC class II clone M5/114.15.2, and Armenian hamster anti-mouse CD11c clone N418.
6. To amplify the antibody signal, incubate each section with biotin-labeled secondary antibodies: use 1:1000 anti-rat IgG and anti-hamster IgG secondary antibodies, and HRP-conjugated avidin for 30 min at room temperature. To detect the antibody signal, employ a substrate/chromogen mixture consisting of 3,30-diaminobenzidine (DAB), followed by hematoxylin counterstaining.
7. Observe the immunostained slides at 20× magnification under bright light, by a photomicroscope equipped with a digital camera (Fig. 2). Capture at least three images from each slide. Pay attention in selecting photos taken under the same lighting conditions.
8. Analyze the image data by using an Imaging software (*see* **Note 10**).
9. For each immunohistochemical stain, choose five to nine fields (width: 58.254 square pixels corresponding to 384355.606 mm^2) per experimental group. Consider the extension of the stained areas in a photographic field as an indicator of the number of stained cells.
10. Detect the stained areas by color-thresholding the image. Measure the resulting area in square pixels.

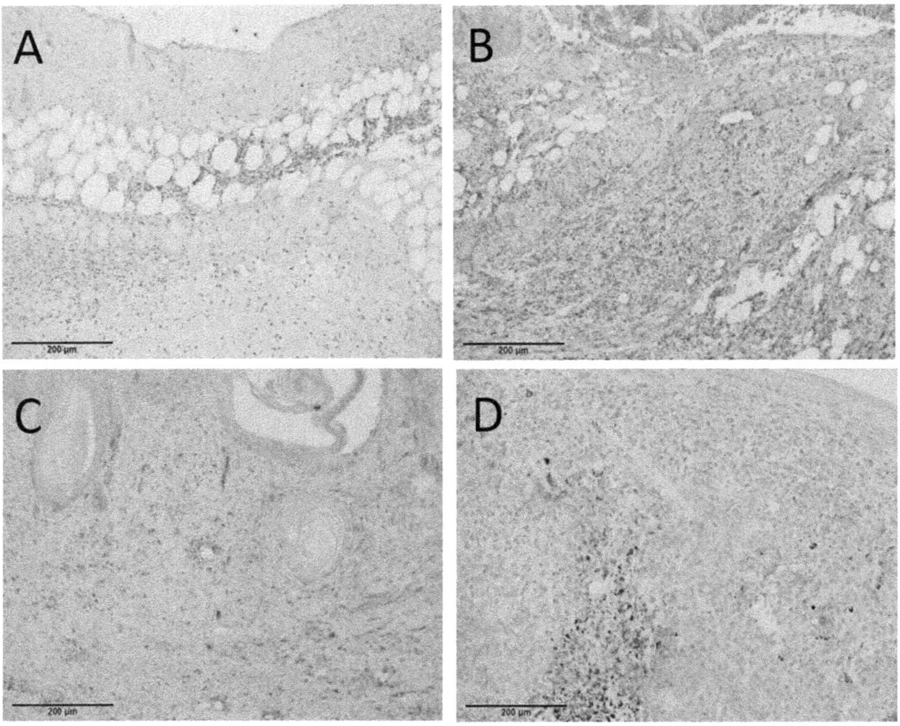

Fig. 2 Representative images of mouse melanoma 7 days after LPS injection. FFPE sections stained with F4/80 (**b**), MHCII (**c**), and CD11c (**d**). In the negative control, the primary antibody has been omitted (**a**). 20× magnification

4 Notes

1. In this study, we used rat anti-mouse F4/80 (clone BM8, eBioscience, San Diego CA, USA) and rat anti-mouse MHCII (clone M5/114.15.2, eBioscience) primary antibodies.
2. In this study, we used Armenian hamster anti-mouse CD11c (clone N418, e Bioscience) primary antibody.
3. In this study, we used anti-rat IgG and anti-hamster IgG secondary antibodies (Invitrogen/Life Technologies).
4. In this study, we used ABC Staining Kit (sc-2019, Santa Cruz).
5. In this study, we used eclipse E600 photomicroscope equipped with a DMX1200 digital camera (Nikon Instruments).
6. Due to possible irritation of the skin, animals should be shaved one or two days before the treatment.
7. Be sure that the cell suspension is thoroughly mixed before you put it into the syringe.

8. The injection of the cell suspension into the subcutaneous region should be done slowly and with no movement of the syringe to ensure the growth of spherical tumors.
9. It is recommended to adjust both image saturation and brightness to exclude the background color.
10. Public domain software for processing and analyzing scientific images—ImageJ software: https://imagej.nih.gov/ij/.

References

1. Talmadge JE, Singh RK, Fidler IJ, Raz A (2007) Murine models to evaluate novel and conventional therapeutic strategies for cancer. Am J Pathol 170:793–804. https://doi.org/10.2353/ajpath.2007.060929
2. Vogelstein B, Papadopoulos N, Velculescu VE, Zhou S, Diaz LA Jr, Kinzler KW (2013) Cancer genome landscapes. Science 339:1546–1558. https://doi.org/10.1126/science.1235122
3. Lee SH, Hong JH, Park HK, Park JS, Kim BK, Lee JY, Jeong JY, Yoon GS, Inoue M, Choi GS, Lee IK (2015) Colorectal cancer-derived tumor spheroids retain the characteristics of original tumors. Cancer Lett 367:34–42. https://doi.org/10.1016/j.canlet.2015.06.024
4. Invrea F, Rovito R, Torchiaro E, Petti C, Isella C, Medico E (2020) Patient-derived xenografts (PDXs) as model systems for human cancer. Curr Opin Biotechnol 63:151–156. https://doi.org/10.1016/j.copbio.2020.01.003
5. Wang M, Yao L-C, Cheng M, Cai D, Martinek J, Pan C-X et al (2018) Humanized mice in studying efficacy and mechanisms of PD-1-targeted cancer immunotherapy. FASEB 32:1537–1549. https://doi.org/10.1096/fj.201700740R
6. Jangalwe S, Shultz LD, Mathew A, Brehm MA (2016) Improved B cell development in humanized NOD-scid IL2Rγ(null) mice transgenically expressing human stem cell factor, granulocyte-macrophage colony-stimulating factor and interleukin-3. Immun Inflamm Dis 4:427–440. https://doi.org/10.1002/iid3.124
7. Lucas ML, Heller L, Coppola D, Heller R (2002) IL-12 plasmid delivery by in vivo electroporation for the successful treatment of established subcutaneous B16.F10 melanoma. Mol Ther 5:668–675
8. Lampreht Tratar U, Loiacono L, Cemazar M, Kamensek U, Fazio VM, Sersa G, Signori E (2017) Gene electrotransfer of plasmid-encoding IL-12 recruits the M1 macrophages and antigen-presenting cells inducing the eradication of aggressive B16F10 murine melanoma. Mediat Inflamm 2017:5285890. https://doi.org/10.1155/2017/5285890
9. Komel T, Bosnjak M, Kranjc Brezar S, De Robertis M, Mastrodonato M, Scillitani G, Pesole G, Signori E, Sersa G, Cemazar M (2021) Gene electrotransfer of IL-2 and IL-12 plasmids effectively eradicated murine B16.F10 melanoma. Bioelectrochemistry 141:107843. https://doi.org/10.1016/j.bioelechem.2021.107843

Chapter 15

Immunospot Assessment of T-Cell Responses in Preclinical Tumor Models with Undefined Target Antigens

Urška Kamenšek and Tinkara Remic

Abstract

Assessment of functional tumor-specific T-cell responses in preclinical tumor models represents an important tool for successful translation of new immunotherapies to clinics. Usually, it requires a known tumor antigen target. Here, we describe the method to detect tumor-specific T cell after immunotherapies without a known antigen. Splenocytes, lymph node immune cells, or PBMCs are isolated from treated mice and stimulated with relevant tumor cells ex vivo before immunospot analysis of Granzyme B and interferon γ-positive T cells. The method is especially valuable for monitoring tumor-specific T cells after vaccination with various whole tumor vaccines or after in situ vaccination and other antigen agnostic immunotherapies, where no specific antigens are used.

Key words Tumor-specific, T cells, Immunospot, FluoroSpot, Granzyme B, Interferon γ, Antigen agnostic immunotherapy, Undefined target antigens

1 Introduction

New immunotherapeutic treatments are constantly being developed and tested in preclinical cancer models. Their desired outcome is to induce a potent T-cell response, which specifically recognizes and eliminates tumor cells. Therefore, robust methods to assess functional tumor-specific T-cell responses in preclinical tumor models are critical for translation of these new treatments into the clinical setting.

Several methods have been introduced to identify tumor-specific T cells [1, 2]. These include antigen-specific tetramer staining assays and interferon γ (IFNγ) immunospot assays that can provide information regarding the frequency and the functionality of antigen specific T cells, but not their cytotoxic potential. Immunospot assays that simultaneously detect both IFNγ and Granzyme B (GrB) secretion may represent a more direct analysis, since GrB is the key mediator of target cell apoptosis by cytotoxic T and natural

Maja Čemažar, Tanja Jesenko and Urša Lampreht Tratar (eds.), *Mouse Models of Cancer: Methods and Protocols*, Methods in Molecular Biology, vol. 2773, https://doi.org/10.1007/978-1-0716-3714-2_15,
© The Author(s), under exclusive license to Springer Science+Business Media, LLC, part of Springer Nature 2024

killer (NK) cells. In a classical enzyme-linked immunospot assay (ELISpot), cells are incubated on the precoated plates (usually 96-well) and allowed to react to any presented stimuli (usually an antigen) to secrete the target protein. The secreted proteins are captured by specific antibodies and made visible by enzyme conjugates. Single cells that produce the target protein form spots that can be visualized and counted on automated immunospot readers or a standard stereomicroscope. FluoroSpot is an adaptation of ELISpot assay that utilizes fluorescent probes instead of enzyme conjugates; thus, enabling multiplex analyses of several analytes secreted by the same cell [3].

Both tetramer and immunospot techniques are antigen-specific, meaning they require a defined antigen target. This presents an issue as antigens are often unknown in preclinical tumor models. Alternatively, surrogate transgenes like ovalbumin (OVA) can be stably introduced to tumor cell lines [4]; however, this can alter the immunogenicity of the preclinical tumor model. Therefore, assays based on recognition of native tumor cells may be more clinically relevant than assays that relay on recognition of a specific tumor antigen. As tumor cells used to generate preclinical tumor models already contain relevant tumor antigens, they can serve as the antigen source for detecting tumor-specific T-cell responses without the need to predefine a target tumor antigen [5, 6].

Here, we describe our method to asses tumor-specific responses after immunotherapies without a known antigen target [7, 8]. FluoroSpot analysis is performed on lymphocytes isolated from lymph nodes of the treated mouse that are cocultured with relevant tumor cells (Fig. 1). The number of dual spot-forming cells corresponds directly to tumor-reactive lymphocytes.

The described method can be employed for other sources of immune cells, such as splenocytes and peripheral blood mononuclear cells (PBMCs). As blood sampling is nonlethal and FluoroSpot is a remarkably sensitive method that can measure responses with frequencies well below 0.0001%, T-cell responses can be examined during the course of treatment and can be correlated with tumor growth delay and survival. Additionally, isolated immune cells can be labeled with fluorescent cell tracers ex vivo and used for adoptive transfer into recipient animals where they can be tracked by intravital imaging (*see* Chap. 13). They can also be used in various T-cell killing assays to directly prove their cytotoxic activity [9, 10].

The method described here is well-suited to study tumor-specific T-cell responses in preclinical tumor models after immunotherapies, particularly after antigen-agnostic immunotherapies, where antigens are not predefined or known, like in situ vaccination or whole tumor cell vaccines.

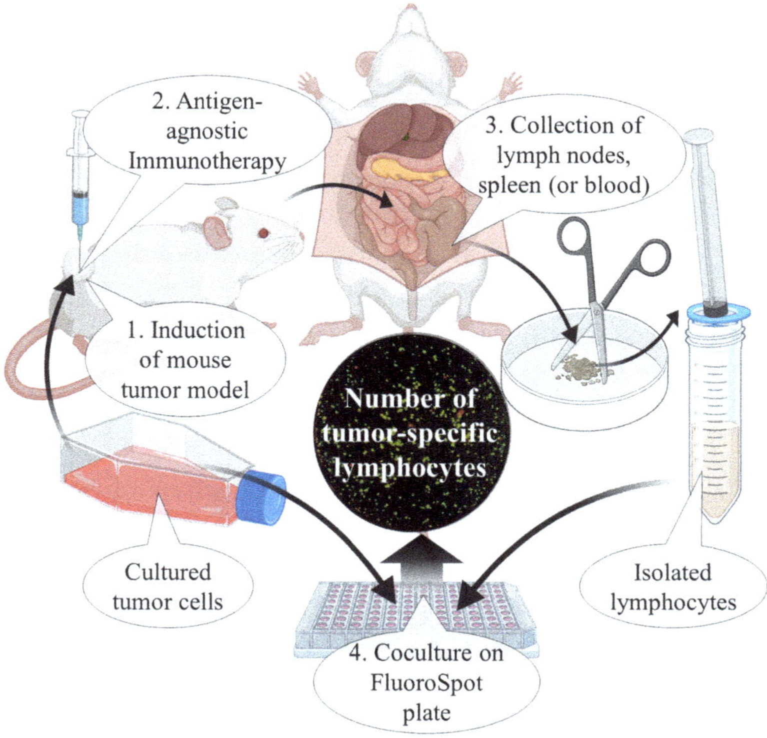

Fig. 1 Ex vivo assessment of tumor-specific T-cell responses by FluoroSpot assay after antigen-agnostic immunotherapy

2 Materials

2.1 Lymphocyte Isolation

1. Treated mice (*see* **Note 1**).
2. Fine surgical tools for animal research.
3. Sterile cell strainer with a 50 μm mesh.
4. Syringe plunger.
5. Chilled phosphate-buffered saline (PBS) (4 °C).
6. Ice.
7. 15 mL centrifuge tubes.
8. Centrifuge for 15 mL tubes.
9. Chilled serum-free freezing media.
10. −20 °C, −80 °C freezers and a freezing container (optional).
11. Laminar flow cabinet/Tissue culture hood.

2.2 Sample Thawing and Cell Recovery

1. Frozen lymphocyte suspensions in cryovials (*see* **Note 2**).
2. Roswell Park Memorial Institute (RPMI) 1640 medium with 4-(2-hydroxyethyl)-1-piperazineethanesulfonic acid (HEPES) + 10% fetal bovine serum (FBS) + 1% Penicillin/Streptomycin + 1% L-glutamine (GlutaMax).

3. DNase I.
4. Hank's Balanced Salt Solution (HBSS) + Ca^{+}+ Mg^{+}.
5. Trypan blue.
6. 15 mL and 50 mL centrifuge tubes.
7. Automatic cell counter or a hemocytometer and a light microscope.
8. Automatic pipettes with tips.
9. Serological pipette with serological pipettes.
10. Water bath (37 °C).
11. Cell incubator (humidified, 37 °C, CO_2).

2.3 FluoroSpot and Data Analysis

1. An ELISpot or FluoroSpot kit (*see* **Note 3**) which includes:
   (a) Membrane-bottom plates.
   (b) Capture antibodies.
   (c) Detection antibodies.
   (d) Dilution buffers for detection antibodies.
   (e) Wash buffer.
   (f) Fluorescence enhancer.
2. Thawed and recovered lymphocytes.
3. Viable tumor cells for stimulation (*see* **Note 4**).
4. Appropriate cell medium for tumor cells.
5. Optional: recombinant IFNγ to prestimulate expression of MHC I on tumor cells (*see* **Note 5**).
6. Deionized water (dH_2O).
7. 35% ethanol or 35% methanol.
8. PBS buffer: 137 mM NaCl, 2.7 mM KCl, 8.1 mM Na_2PO_4. Adjust the pH to 7.4. Use a 0.2 μm filter membrane to filter through the PBS solution before use.
9. Blocking buffer: 1% BSA and 5% sucrose in PBS. Use a 0.2 μm filter membrane to filter through the blocking buffer before use.
10. 500 mL measuring cylinder.
11. Sterile (filtered) RPMI 1640 medium HEPES + 10% FBS + 1% Penicillin/Streptomycin + 1% Glutamax.
12. A conventional epifluorescent microscope or/and ELISpot reader capable of detecting fluorescent signals.
13. Pipettes and appropriate tips (recommended use of multichannel with reagent reservoirs or electronic pipettes).
14. Cell incubator (humidified, 37 °C, CO_2).
15. Laminar flow cabinet/Tissue culture hood.

3 Methods

3.1 Lymphocyte Isolation

Before you start, prepare an aseptic work environment.

1. As soon as the mice are humanely sacrificed, aseptically harvest the draining lymph nodes or the spleen (*see* **Note 6**).
2. Put the harvested tissue into a 60 mm petri dish with 2–3 mL chilled PBS (4 °C).
3. Using sterile surgical scissors, shear the tissue as much as possible.
4. Transfer the tissue onto a 50 μm sterile strainer on a 15 mL centrifuge tube (*see* **Note 7**).
5. Using the rough side of the syringe plunger, mesh the tissue through the strainer to make a single cell suspension.
6. Rinse gradually with chilled PBS up to the final volume of 10 mL.
7. Centrifuge for 5 min at 500 × *g*, 4 °C, and discard the supernatant.
8. Wash the pellet with 5 mL of chilled PBS.
9. When isolating lymphocytes from spleen, we recommend an additional step for lysis of erythrocytes. This can be performed using a commercially available lysing buffer, after the **step 8**.
10. Centrifuge for 5 min at 500 × *g*, 4 °C, and discard the supernatant.
11. Resuspend the pellet in 1–2 mL of chilled serum-free freezing Media (4 °C) (*see* **Note 8**) and transfer 1 mL into an appropriately marked cryovial.
12. After an overnight incubation at −20 °C (*see* **Note 9**), store the lymphocytes at −80 °C for future analysis. The lymphocytes should be used within a month from freezing for optimal results.

3.2 Sample Thawing

Once all your samples are collected and you are ready to proceed with ELISpot/FluoroSpot analysis, thaw your samples as needed. Avoid multiple thaw-freeze cycles.

1. Take the selected samples from −80 °C and shortly incubate in a water bath at 37 °C until the walls of the cryovials are thawed.
2. Wipe the cryovials carefully with ethanol and under sterile conditions slowly add 1 mL of prewarmed RPMI-1640 medium with HEPES (37 °C).
3. Transfer the cell suspension into 8 mL of warm RPMI-1640 medium with HEPES contained in 50 mL centrifuge tubes.

4. Centrifuge for 10 min at 500 × *g* at room temperature and carefully discard the supernatant.
5. Resuspend the cell pellet in 2 mL of prewarmed HBSS + Ca^+ + Mg^+) (37 °C).
6. Add DNase I at 2 U/mL (*see* **Note 10**).
7. Incubate at 37 °C with shaking (200 rpm) for 45 min.
8. Count the cells using a hemocytometer or an automatic cell counter (*see* **Note 11**).
9. Add prewarmed RPMI-1640 medium with HEPES until the concentration reaches 2×10^6 cells/mL.
10. Allow cells to recover overnight in a humidified 37 °C CO_2 incubator with loosened caps.

3.3 FluoroSpot

Depending on the ELISpot or FluoroSpot assay, the process spans 3–5 days and begins on the same day as sample thawing. Before you start, plate the tumor cells you intend to use for stimulation of lymphocytes so that they will be 80% confluent at the day of stimulation (day 2) (*see* **Note 12**).

Before you begin each day, bring all the necessary reagents to room temperature.

Day 1: FluoroSpot plate preparation

1. Prepare the plate according to the instructions provided in the kit. The steps include prewetting (*see* **Note 13**), incubation, rinsing (*see* **Note 14**), and the addition of capture antibodies.
2. Incubate overnight at 2–8 °C.

Day 2: Sample addition and stimulation

1. Continue according to the instructions provided in the kit. The steps include rinsing, addition of blocking buffer, incubation, and replacement of blocking buffer with RPMI-1640 medium with HEPES.
2. Add your samples and stimulant: empty the wells and add a total of 100 μL of the necessary controls (*see* **Note 15**) as well as the optimized ratio of lymphocytes and the stimulant, i.e., tumor cells, in RPMI-1640 medium with HEPES.
3. Incubate for 48 h in a humidified 37 °C CO_2 incubator (*see* **Note 16**).

Day 4: Addition of the first detection antibody

1. According to the instructions provided in the kit, rinse the plate and add the first (fluorescent) detection antibody (e.g., IFNγ) (*see* **Note 17**).
2. Incubate overnight at 2–8 °C (*see* **Note 18**).

Day 5: Addition of the second detection antibody

1. According to the instructions provided in the kit, rinse the plate and add the second detection antibody (e.g., GrB) (*see* **Note 17**) and incubate. If the kit incorporates a fluorescent enhancer, add it to the plate after rinsing the second detection antibody.
2. Remove the underdrain and leave the plate to dry in the dark.

3.4 Data Analysis

1. Once dry (24 h), the wells may be imaged and analyzed using an ELISpot reader capable of detecting fluorescent signals or with a conventional epifluorescent microscope (*see* **Note 19**).
2. Using an image processing software, i.e., Image J, overlay images of the wells taken using appropriate excitation emission wavelengths.
3. Count the spots positive for each antibody (green and red) and double positive (yellow).
4. Subtract the number of double positive spots gained from wells with unstimulated lymphocytes (N_{Unstimul}) from the number of double positive spots gained from wells with stimulated lymphocytes (N_{Stimul}). With this formula, you avoid including nonspecific effector lymphocytes:

$$N_{\mathrm{TS}} = N_{\mathrm{Stimul}} - N_{\mathrm{Unstimul}}$$

   This number of spots positive for both GrB and IFNγ corresponds to the number of tumor-specific (N_{TS}) lymphocytes (Fig. 2).
5. Lastly, data can be presented as the fold-change relative to tumor-specific lymphocytes present in the untreated/mock-treated control group.

4 Notes

1. Mice with induced tumors (syngeneic mouse tumor model) treated with the selected immunotherapy serve as a source of lymphocytes, which are isolated at a specific time point after treatment and used for the immunospot assay (Fig. 1). In our study, we used the B16F10 tumor model syngeneic to C57BL/6 mice and the CT26 tumor model syngeneic to BALB/c mice. We isolated the lymphocytes from the lymph nodes 6 days after the treatment [7].
2. In our experiments, we used frozen lymphocytes isolated from the draining lymph nodes of the treated mice. However, depending on the experimental aims, fresh or frozen

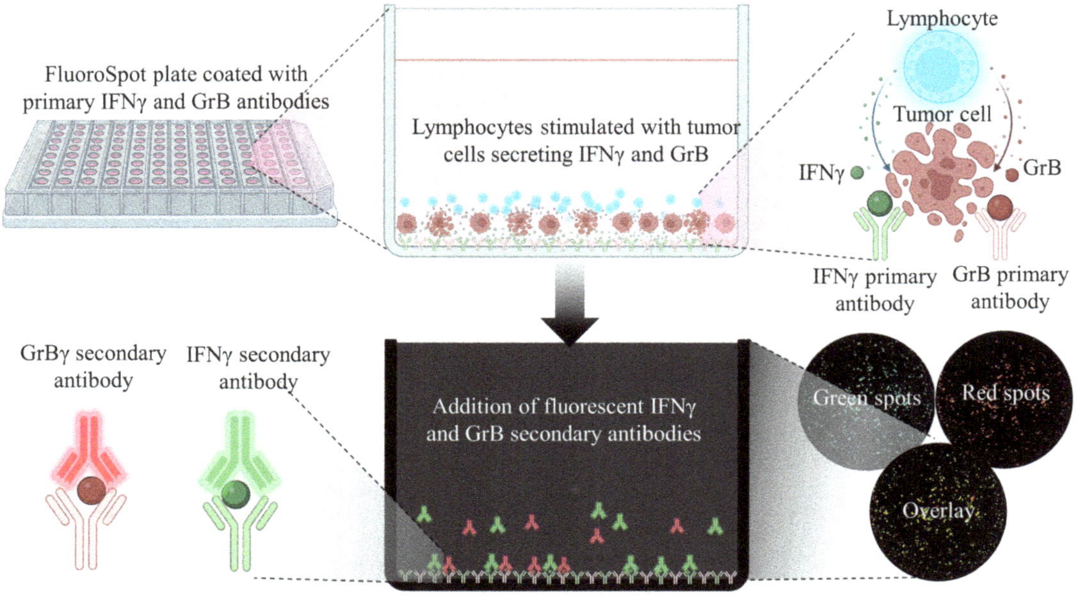

Fig. 2 FluoroSpot assay with tumor cells stimulating effector lymphocytes to secrete IFNγ and GrB

lymphocytes isolated from spleen, blood, or lymph nodes can also be used [11–13]. Different methods of cryopreservation and lymphocytes recovery can impact the results [14, 15].

3. We used the R&D Systems Mouse IFN-gamma/Granzyme B Dual-Color FluoroSpot Kit (ELD5819NL, R&D Systems, USA).
4. Use tumors cells that were used to induce the preclinical tumor model on which you tested your treatment (Fig. 1). These cells contain relevant tumor antigens and serve as antigen source for the detection of tumor-specific T-cell responses. In our study, we used B16F10 and CT26 tumor cells [7].
5. rIFNγ can be used to induce the expression of MHC I molecules on cancer cell lines (especially B16F10 with inherently low MHC I expression), enabling them to present tumor antigens to T cells [6]. In our experiments, we chose not to use rIFNy to simulate a more accurate in vivo situation. Furthermore, IFNy should already be secreted by the immune cells plated with the tumor cells.
6. In our experiments, we harvested the draining lymph nodes, as they are an important site of interaction between tumor borne antigens, antigen-presenting cells, and lymphocytes, and may best represent the initial stages of the systemic immune response [16].
7. To increase cell viability, work on ice, especially when working with a larger number of samples.

8. To increase cell viability after thawing, we recommend suspending 10^6 cells in 1 mL of media, but no more than 5×10^6 cells per 1 mL of media.
9. Alternatively, freezing container, e.g., Mr. Frosty, can be used to slowly freeze the cells.
10. Use DNase I to prevent cell clumping [7, 11]. During thawing, DNA and debris released from ruptured cells can cause clumping and, subsequently loss of cells trapped in the clumps. Especially in FluoroSpot assays, these clumps can prevent effective analysis of lymphocytes immune function.
11. Use Trypan Blue or any other stain to only count the number of live cells for further analysis.
12. The number of lymphocytes and the number of tumor cells used to stimulate the lymphocytes should be optimized. We have successfully used a 1:10 ratio of lymphocytes to tumor cells, i.e., 2×10^5 lymphocytes: 2×10^4 tumor cells.
13. Pay attention to the manufacturer's protocol, as this step depends on the membrane bottom of the plate. If your plate has a PVDF or other hydrophobic membrane bottom, the membrane must be prewetted with 35% ethanol or 35% methanol. Once the wells are prewetted, the membrane must remain wet until the end of the process.
14. Empty the wells by turning the plate over and tapping it against a clean paper towel. Avoid aspirating the liquid with a pipette tip as this may damage the membrane.
15. The controls should be the positive (recombinant IFNγ or recombinant GrB), negative (unstimulated lymphocytes and tumor cells only), stimulant only, background (e.g., sterile culture media), and detection antibody control (PBS).
16. To avoid evaporation and subsequent drying of the membrane, wrap the covered plate with parafilm.
17. Detection antibodies must be prepared immediately before use.
18. Cover the plate and wrap it with parafilm to prevent evaporation. To prevent edge effect, wrap the plate additionally in aluminum foil.
19. In case of using a conventional epifluorescent microscope, we recommend carefully removing the membrane bottoms with a 6 mm puncher and fixing the membranes on a nonautofluorescent material, e.g., a glass slide.

References

1. Lim KP, Zainal NS (2021) Monitoring T cells responses mounted by therapeutic cancer vaccines. Front Mol Biosci 8. https://doi.org/10.3389/fmolb.2021.623475
2. Malyguine AM, Strobl S, Dunham K, Shurin MR, Sayers TJ (2012) ELISPOT assay for monitoring cytotoxic T lymphocytes (CTL) activity in cancer vaccine clinical trials. Cells 1: 111. https://doi.org/10.3390/cells1020111
3. Janetzki S, Rueger M, Dillenbeck T, Kalyuzhny AE (2014) Stepping up ELISpot: multi-level analysis in FluoroSpot assays. Cell 3:1102. https://doi.org/10.3390/cells3041102
4. Akache B, McCluskie MJ (2021) The quantification of antigen-specific t cells by IFN-γ elispot. Methods Mol Biol. https://doi.org/10.1007/978-1-0716-0795-4_30
5. van Vloten JP, Santry LA, McAusland TM, Karimi K, McFadden G, Petrik JJ, Wootton SK, Bridle BW (2019) Quantifying antigen-specific T cell responses when using antigen-agnostic immunotherapies. Mol Ther Methods Clin Dev 13:154. https://doi.org/10.1016/j.omtm.2019.01.012. PMID: 30788384; PMCID: PMC6369252
6. Malyguine A, Strobl SL, Shafer-Weaver KA, Ulderich T, Troke A, Baseler M, Kwak LW, Neelapu SS (2004) A modified human ELISPOT assay to detect specific responses to primary tumor cell targets. J Transl Med 2. https://doi.org/10.1186/1479-5876-2-9
7. Remic T, Sersa G, Levpuscek K, Lampreht Tratar U, Ursic Valentinuzzi K, Cör A, Kamensek U (2022) Tumor cell-based vaccine contributes to local tumor irradiation by eliciting a tumor model-dependent systemic immune response. Front Immunol 13. https://doi.org/10.3389/fimmu.2022.974912
8. Kamensek U, Cemazar M, Lampreht Tratar U, Ursic K, Sersa G (2018) Antitumor in situ vaccination effect of TNFα and IL-12 plasmid DNA electrotransfer in a murine melanoma model. Cancer Immunol Immunother 67: 785. https://doi.org/10.1007/s00262-018-2133-0. Epub 2018 Feb 21
9. Graef P, Buchholz VR, Busch DH (2010) Killer cell assays. Methods Microbiol. https://doi.org/10.1016/S0580-9517(10)37008-5
10. Matta H, Gopalakrishnan R, Choi S et al (2018) Development and characterization of a novel luciferase based cytotoxicity assay. Sci Rep 8:199. https://doi.org/10.1038/s41598-017-18606-1
11. García-Piñeres AJ, Hildesheim A, Williams M, Trivett M, Strobl S, Pinto LA (2006) DNase treatment following thawing of cryopreserved PBMC is a procedure suitable for lymphocyte functional studies. J Immunol Methods 313: 209. https://doi.org/10.1016/j.jim.2006.04.004. Epub 2006 May 17
12. Santos R, Buying A, Sabri N, Yu J, Gringeri A, Bender J, Janetzki S, Pinilla C, Judkowski VA (2015) Improvement of IFNg ELISPOT performance following overnight resting of frozen PBMC samples confirmed through rigorous statistical analysis. Cells 4:1. https://doi.org/10.3390/cells4010001
13. Mallone R, Mannering SI, Brooks-Worrell BM, Durinovic-Belló I, Cilio CM, Wong FS, Schloot NC (2011) Isolation and preservation of peripheral blood mononuclear cells for analysis of islet antigen-reactive T cell responses: position statement of the T-Cell Workshop Committee of the Immunology of Diabetes Society. Clin Exp Immunol 163:33. https://doi.org/10.1111/j.1365-2249.2010.04272.x. Epub 2010 Oct 5
14. Gad E, Rastetter L, Herendeen D, Curtis B, Slota M, Koehnlein M, Disis N (2013) Optimizing the cryopreservation of murine splenocytes for improved antigen-specific T cell function in ELISPOT. J Immunother Cancer 1. https://doi.org/10.1186/2051-1426-1-S1-P211
15. Maecker HT, Moon J, Bhatia S et al (2005) Impact of cryopreservation on tetramer, cytokine flow cytometry, and ELISPOT. BMC Immunol 6. https://doi.org/10.1186/1471-2172-6-17
16. Buchwald ZS, Nasti TH, Lee J, Eberhardt CS, Wieland A, Im SJ, Lawson D, Curran W, Ahmed R, Khan MK (2020) Tumor-draining lymph node is important for a robust abscopal effect stimulated by radiotherapy. J Immunother Cancer 8:e000867. https://doi.org/10.1136/jitc-2020-000867

Chapter 16

Necropsy in Mouse Research

Snježana Čužić, Vuk Milutinović, Maja Antolić, and Anja Ognjenović

Abstract

Necropsy is the postmortem examination of an animal's body. Experiments on laboratory animals are performed to gather scientific data relevant to basic and, even more often, translational research, mainly in the field of translational medicine. A necropsy conducted on laboratory animals subjected to experimental research provides an opportunity to exhaustively explore pathological processes that took place during life. In order to achieve that goal, procedures of biomaterial collection should be performed timely, bearing in mind the inevitable process of postmortem tissue decay, and precisely, to avoid mechanical tissue damage.

In this chapter, procedures of collecting organs and tissue in a way that ensures the preservation of the organ structure, tissue organization, morphological characteristics of cells, and last but not least, intracellular protein and nucleic acid content and chromosome organization are going to be described step by step.

Key words Laboratory animal, Mouse, Necropsy, Protocol, Research, Translational medicine, Oncology

1 Introduction

Postmortem examination of the body is performed to determine the cause of death, evaluate the character and extension of pathohistological changes, as well as to define the disease's etiology and pathophysiology. A postmortem examination performed on an animal body is called necropsy [1]. During necropsy, all observed macroscopic changes, i.e., visible by the naked eye, are noted and tissue and organ samples are stored for further evaluation using various techniques.

The aim of this chapter is to describe necropsy techniques used in experimental work on mice in the spirit of Replacement, Reduction and Refinement (3R). Ethical principles of 3R [2] are set, among others, to reduce the number of animals needed to obtain reliable and relevant scientific data. In order to achieve the aim of 3R, researchers are encouraged to meticulously plan sample collection from experimental animals engaged in the study [3].

Maja Čemažar, Tanja Jesenko and Urša Lampreht Tratar (eds.), *Mouse Models of Cancer: Methods and Protocols*, Methods in Molecular Biology, vol. 2773, https://doi.org/10.1007/978-1-0716-3714-2_16,
© The Author(s), under exclusive license to Springer Science+Business Media, LLC, part of Springer Nature 2024

In the authors' eyes, necropsy should be performed on naïve and challenged animals enrolled in the experiment. During necropsy, target organ(s)/tissue, and those playing a role in the model's pathophysiological pathway need to be collected. To further optimize sample collection, the biomaterial is to be preserved appropriately to enable a wide range of subsequent analyses performed immediately after cessation of *in life* phase or with a delay.

2 Materials

To successfully perform the necropsy, one should prepare the following.

2.1 Equipment

1. Protective clothing, eyeglasses, rubber gloves, and mask.
2. Styrofoam dissection board (15 × 15 cm, 3 cm thick) wrapped in aluminum wrapping foil.
3. Cork boards (3 × 3 cm, 3 mm thick).
4. Blunt forceps of various sizes (pointed and serrated forceps should be avoided since they can damage the tissue).
5. Surgical scissors of various sizes.
6. Round-end enterotomy scissors.
7. Syringes (1 mL, 2 mL, 5 mL, and 10 mL).
8. Needles of various sizes (27 G is used for instilling fixative into the lungs).
9. Straight, inflexible oral gavage needle.
10. Scalpels (with exchangeable blades of various sizes and shapes).
11. Single-edge razorblade.
12. Surgical curette spoon.
13. Surgical suturing material.
14. Marked containers filled up to two-third with fixative, 500 mL, 750 mL, or 1000 mL in volume, allowing the tissue to fixative volume ratio of 1:50.
15. Specific containers for other types of samples (hematology, virology, microbiology).
16. Plastic Petri dishes.
17. Labeled cassettes for histopathological processing.
18. Precision scale.
19. Depilation cream.
20. Single-use shaving razor.
21. Digital camera.
22. Necropsy recording sheets.

2.2 Solutions

1. 10% neutral-buffered formalin (NBF): 4% *formaldehyde solution.*
2. Davidson's fixative: 2 parts of 10% neutral buffered formalin, 3 parts of Ethanol absolute 99.9%, 1-part Acetic acid (glacial) 100%, 3 parts tap water.
3. Decalcifying solution: 9 parts 10% neutral-buffered formalin, 1-part *formic acid.*
4. Cold Phosphate Buffer Solution (PBS): 0.0027 M potassium chloride, 0.137 M sodium chloride, pH 7.4.
5. 70% and 95% Ethanol.
6. 0.9% saline solution: 0.9% NaCl in sterilized water.

3 Methods

3.1 External Examination

After euthanasia and exsanguination of the animal through the external jugular vein (*see* **Note 1**), an external examination is performed. Assess the general condition of the animal and record any external changes (skin lesions, changes of the skin color, fur loss or discoloration, and subcutaneous masses) describing their exact localization and gross appearance. Examine the mucosal surface of all orifices (conjunctival, oral, nasal, anogenital) and record any abnormalities.

3.2 Integumentary System and Mammary Glands

Place the animal ventral side up onto the dissection board. Extend the neck, tail, and all of the limbs, and affix them to the dissection board using five 21 G needles (*see* **Note 2**). Moisten the hair on the ventral side of the animal using 70% ethanol (Fig. 1a).

Examine the mammary glands. Mice have five pairs of mammary glands, three thoracic and two abdominal, and mammary gland tissue is diffusely distributed lateral to the midline, on both sides. The inguinal region is the preferred region for sampling in

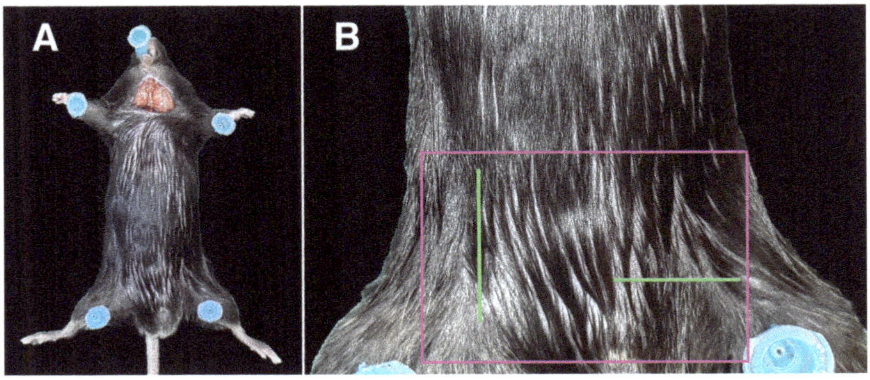

Fig. 1 (**a**) Animal affixed to the dissection board. (**b**) Sampling directions of the mammary glands

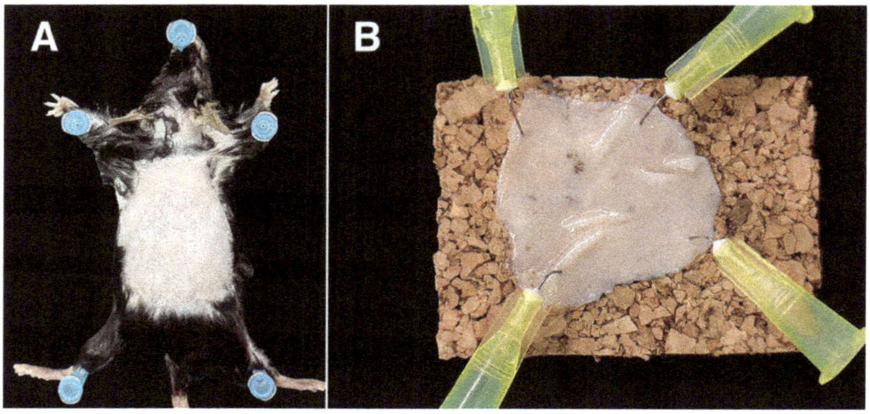

Fig. 2 (**a**) Shaven region of the skin for sampling. (**b**) Skin sample affixed to the corkboard

both males and females. Samples can be taken longitudinally or transversally in a 1 × 3 cm area (Fig. 1b) along with the skin and nipples. Prior to sampling, in order to achieve a better quality of the samples, trimming or shaving of the hair is recommended.

For a sampling of a larger skin area, the animal should be placed dorsal side up onto the dissection board, and using an epilation crème and a single-use shaving razor, desired area of the skin should be shaved (Fig. 2a). After shaving, cut the surface of the skin using a surgical blade in the required shape. Using blunt forceps, grab and pull on one of the edges, and by surgical blade cut the subcutaneous tissue in order to separate the skin. After dissection, place the skin onto a cork board, epidermal face down, stretch, and affix it to the board using several 21 G needles (Fig. 2b). Place the sample into a formalin-filled container sample side down (*see* **Note 3**).

3.3 Opening of the Abdominal Cavity and Sampling of the Abdominal Organs

3.3.1 Gastrointestinal Tract

With the animal positioned ventral side up on the dissection board, the skin incision is made along the midline, stretching from the pubis to the mandible. In male animals, the incision should end on both sides of the penis (Fig. 3a). Fold back the skin on both sides of the incision and affix it to the dissection board using needles. Examine the skin and the subcutaneous tissue, recording all lesions. Observe and record the amount of subcutaneous fat tissue, color and developmental status of muscle tissue, and presence, location, and size of subcutaneous lymph nodes.

Open the abdominal cavity with a longitudinal incision along the midline, stretching from the xiphoid process of the sternum to the pelvis, making sure not to cut any of the intra-abdominal organs (*see* **Note 4**). Fold back the abdominal wall on both sides. Abdominal muscles are sampled using blunt forceps and surgical scalpels or scissors.

Move the intestine of the animal to its right side. The spleen is an elongated, oval, slightly curved reddish organ situated in the upper left abdominal quadrant. It is surrounded by connective and

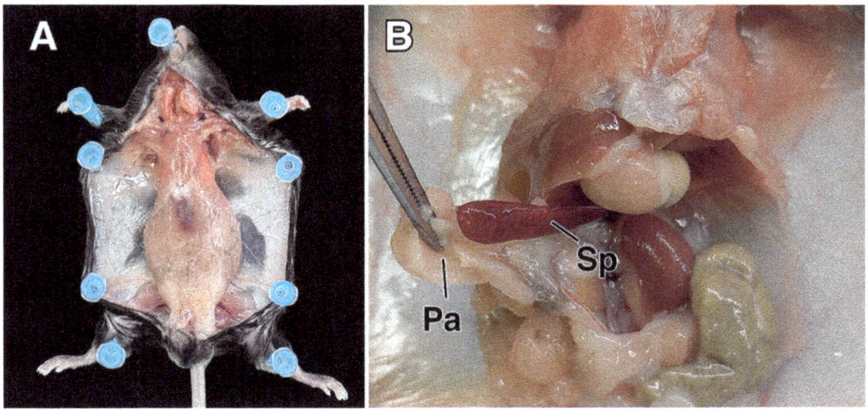

Fig. 3 (**a**) Midline incision from the mandible to the pubic region, (**b**) spleen, and pancreas (Sp—spleen, Pa—pancreas)

fat tissue and attached to the stomach with the gastrosplenic ligament. In order to sample it, grab the surrounding fat tissue with blunt forceps. Cut the connective tissue and fat along the hilum, and the gastrosplenic ligament (Fig. 3b).

After removing the spleen, submerge the entire organ in a buffered formalin fixative. The remaining fat tissue surrounding the spleen is also sampled since it contains the pancreas left lobe.

Grasping with blunt forceps onto the fat tissue surrounding the stomach, pull the stomach gently downward, exposing the intra-abdominal part of the esophagus. Cut the esophagus with the scissors, as close as possible to the diaphragm, and continue pulling onto the fat tissue downward and to the left side of the animal. Dissect the fat and connective tissue in order to free the stomach and duodenum. Place the organs on the right side of the animal.

The liver is a large organ situated in the cranial part of the abdomen. It consists of the right medial, right lateral lobe, left lateral, left medial lobe, caudate lobe, and papillary process. The gallbladder is located on the dorsal side of the liver. To remove the liver from the abdominal cavity, grasp and lift the xiphoid process upward with forceps and expose, the liver and its connections to the diaphragm (falciform ligament) (Fig. 4a). Cut the falciform ligament with scissors, paying close attention not to cut into the liver tissue. Grasping the remnants of the ligaments with blunt forceps, extirpate the liver from the abdomen (Fig. 4b). Do not touch liver parenchyma with forceps (*see* **Note 5**). Immerse the liver in a container filled with formalin [4].

After the removal of the liver, the next step is to isolate the intestine. This is achieved by dissecting the skin around the anus, placing the tip of large scissors between the rectum and pelvis, and cutting through the pelvic arch. Grasp the rectum with forceps, separate it from the vagina and uterus in females, and pull it upward

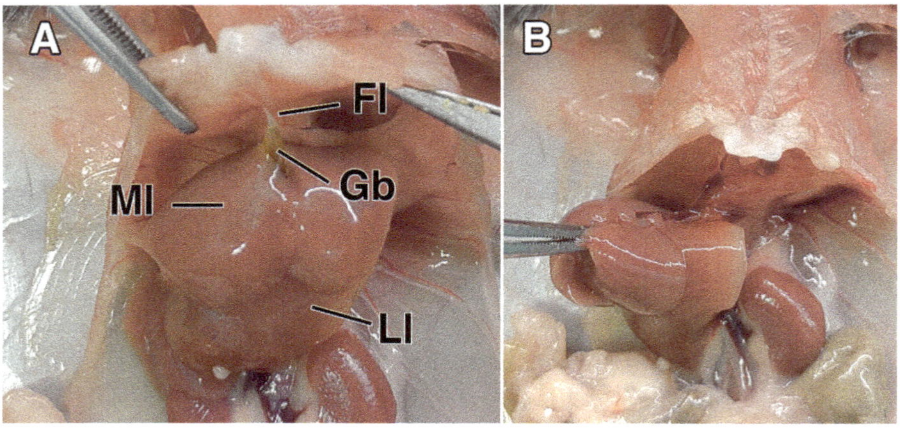

Fig. 4 (**a**) Liver (Ll—left lobe, Ml—medial lobe, Gb—gallbladder, Fl—falciform ligament) and (**b**) extirpation of the liver

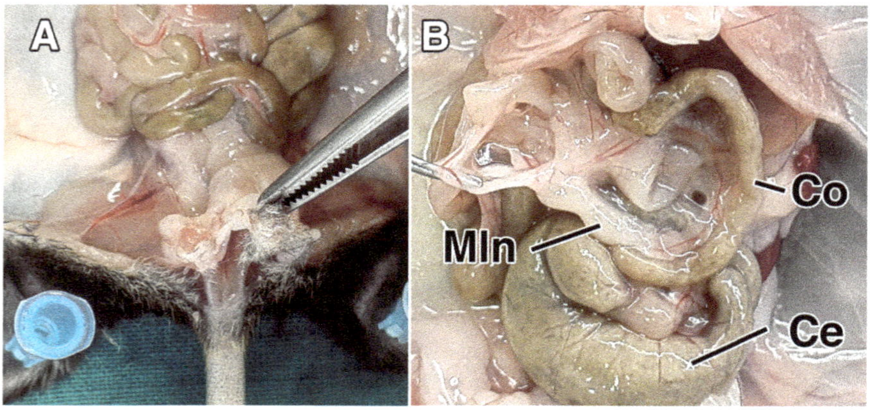

Fig. 5 (**a**) Isolation of the rectum and (**b**) mesenteric lymph nodes (Mln—mesenteric lymph nodes, Ce—cecum, Co—colon)

(Fig. 5a). Continue to gradually extract the intestine in a caudal-cranial direction, while cutting the insertion of the mesentery as close to the intestine as possible. Mesenteric lymph nodes are located within the mesentery, between the cecum, transversal colon, and small intestine (Fig. 5b). They should be sampled, using scissors and forceps, and immediately put in a formalin-filled container.

Upon the removal of the stomach and intestine, separate the stomach together with the duodenum (1 cm) from the rest of the intestine, open the stomach along the greater curvature, empty the content of the stomach, rinse it in cold PBS solution, place it on the corkboard, mucosal side up and fix with four needles (Fig. 6a). Transfer it to a buffered formalin fixative-filled container, paying attention that the tissue is fully immersed (*see* **Note 6**).

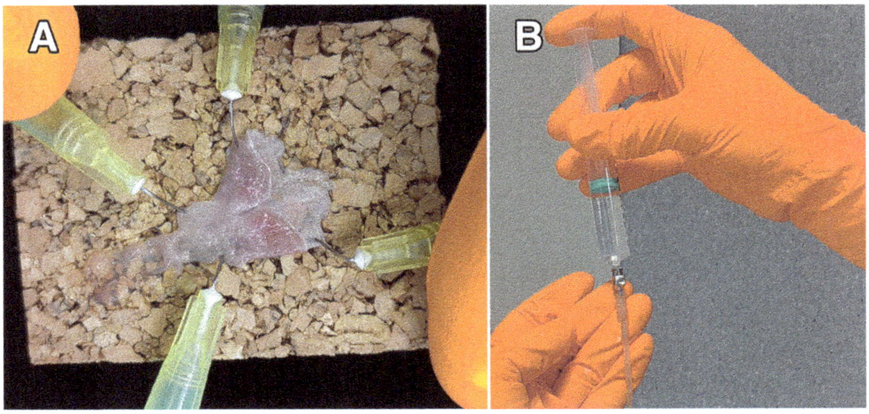

Fig. 6 (**a**) Stomach and (**b**) rinsing of the small intestine

In order to rinse the content from the intestine, separate the small intestine from the large at the insertion point of the small intestine into the cecum. Mount an inflexible oral gavage needle to a large syringe filled with cold PBS solution, and rinse the intestine clear of any content (Fig. 6b). Remove the cecum with a small part of the colon, and rinse the fecal content from the colon in the same way.

3.3.2 Genitourinary Organs

The urinary system consists of kidneys, ureters, and urinary bladder. Extraction of kidneys is performed together with the adrenal glands, which are located at the upper pole of the kidneys and surrounded by fat and connective tissue. Extraction is performed by grasping the periureteral connective tissue at the lower end of a ureter, and pulling it upward (Fig. 7a). Trim the excess fat surrounding the kidneys and isolate both adrenal glands. All the organs are immediately transferred into the container field with a buffered formalin fixative.

Gently grasp the urinary bladder with blunt forceps and pull it upward. Put a surgical ligature at its neck, and fill the bladder with 0.05 mL of formalin (do not instill fixative if the bladder is already distended with urine) (Fig. 7b). Once filled, make a transversal cut across its neck, below the ligature, and transfer it to the buffered formalin-filled container.

The female genital apparatus consists of the uterus, ovaries, oviducts, and vagina situated within the inferior part of the abdominal cavity, adherent to the posterior abdominal wall. The female genital tract is excised by dissecting the skin surrounding the vulva, grasping the vaginal channel with blunt forceps and pulling upward, dissecting the connective and fat tissue surrounding the organs, until they are removed from the abdominal cavity (Fig. 8).

The male genital apparatus consists of testes, epididymis, seminal vesicles, coagulating glands, prostate, and preputial glands. Testes are oval-shaped, paired organs, grayish-white in color with

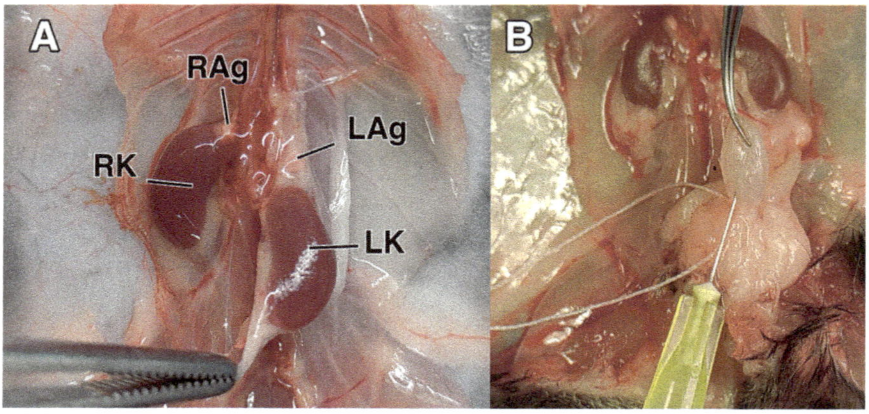

Fig. 7 (**a**) Kidneys and adrenal gland (RK—right kidney, LK—left kidney, RAg—right adrenal gland, LAg—left adrenal gland) and (**b**) urinary bladder

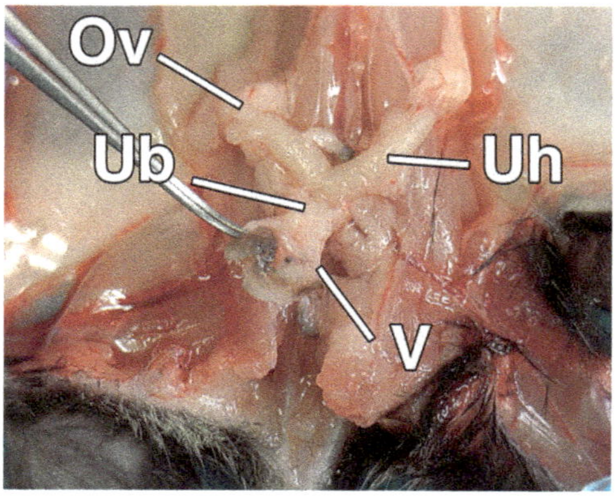

Fig. 8 Uterus and ovaries (V—vagina, Ub—uterus body, Uh—uterus horn, Ov—ovaries)

a soft consistency, located inside the scrotum, or sometimes can be found in the abdominal cavity.

In order to remove the testis, gently grab the inguinal fat pad and cut it away from the abdominal cavity, together with the epididymis (Fig. 9a). After removal, both organs should be placed together into Davidson's fixative for 24 h, followed by fixation in buffered formalin.

Seminal vesicles are curved flattened shaped structures, grey in color, found on both bladder sides, in close relation with coagulating glands, and in communication with the urethra. Remove the group of adjacent organs consisting of the prostate, urinary bladder, seminal vesicles, and coagulating glands in toto, and immerse them in buffered formalin fixative (Fig. 9b).

Preputial glands are located on both sides of the penis. Glands are large, round, and yellow in color. Grasp the gland on one pole with blunt forceps, and dissect it from the surrounding tissue. Transfer the organ to the buffered formalin-filled container.

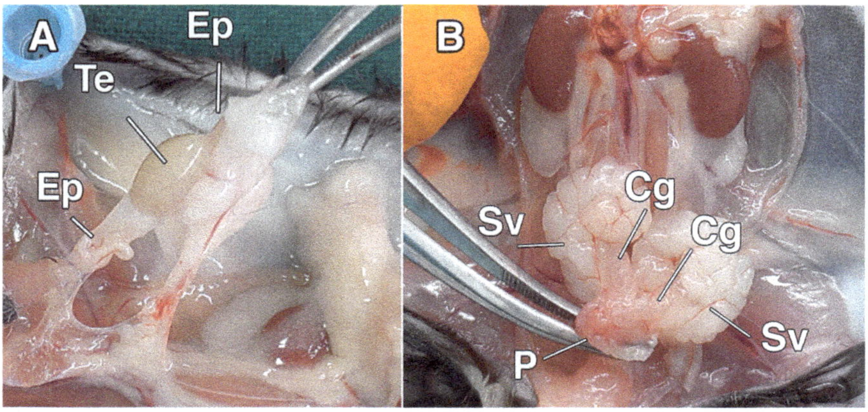

Fig. 9 (**a**) Testis and epididymis (Te—testis, Ep—epididymis), and (**b**) prostate and seminal vesicles (P—prostate, Sv—seminal vesicles, Cg—coagulating glands)

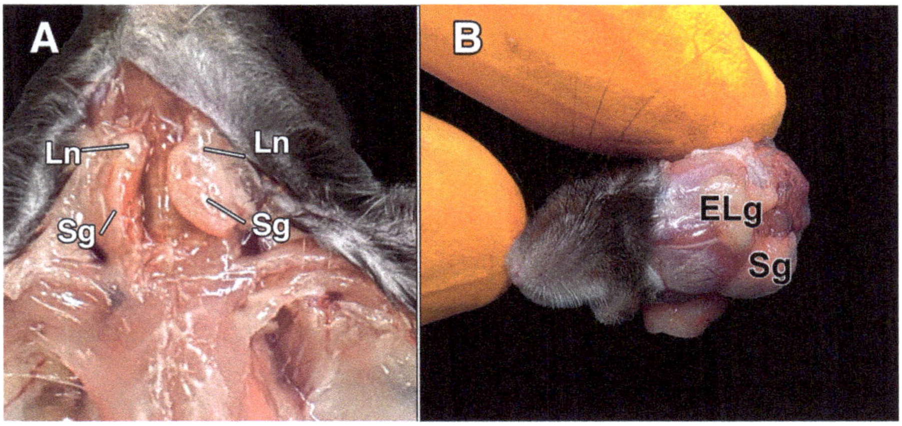

Fig. 10 (**a**) Ventral neck region (Sg—mandibular salivary gland, Ln—mandibular lymph node). (**b**) Extraorbital tear glands (ELg—extraorbital tear gland, Sg—salivary gland)

3.4 Sampling of the Neck Organs

Salivary glands are located on both sides within the cranioventral region of the neck (Fig. 10a). There are three pairs of salivary glands: mandibular, parotid, and sublingual. Remove them together, along with mandibular lymph nodes *en bloc*, by gently grasping the lower tip of the largest salivary gland with forceps. Then, slowly pull toward yourself, cutting the surrounding connective tissues with scissors and immersing the glands in a fixative solution upon removal (Fig. 10a).

The extra orbital lacrimal gland can be removed separately, or together with other glands (salivary glands, mandibular lymph nodes, and parotid gland) (Fig. 10b).

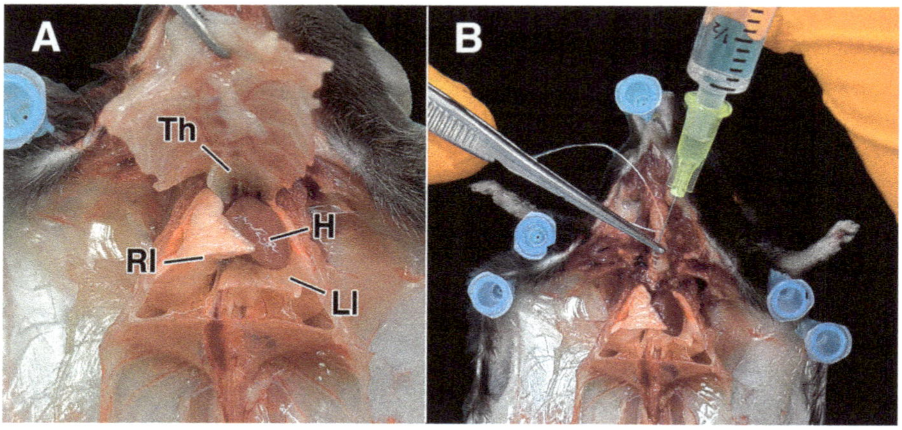

Fig. 11 (**a**) Thoracic cavity (Th—thymus, Rl—right lung, Ll—left lung, H—heart). (**b**) Instillation of formalin into lungs

3.5 Opening of the Thoracic Cavity and Sampling of Thoracic Organs

The thoracic cavity is opened by lifting the xiphoid process with forceps and cutting with scissors from the last rib to the clavicle-sternal articulation, cutting along the line of junction of the rib with sternal cartilage. After cutting the ribs, cut the frontal diaphragm insertion at on the back of the sternum. Place the sternum with a section of the ribs in buffered formalin fixative.

The thymus consists of two lobes and lies in the middle of the thoracic cavity, close to the base of the heart (Fig. 11a). Upon opening the thoracic cavity, isolate the thymus by grabbing the lower part of one of the lobes, and cutting the ligament connecting it to the pericardium.

For optimal microscopic evaluation of the lung parenchyma, the instillation of the lung with 10% buffered formalin is recommended. Attach a 21 G needle to a 2 mL syringe filled with buffered formalin. Isolate the trachea, place a ligature around it and insert the needle into the trachea below the ligature (Fig. 11b). Grasp the trachea, with the needle in it, gently push the plunger of the syringe and fill the lungs with formalin (*see* **Note 7**). Make a transverse cut across the trachea, esophagus, and main vessels in the proximal region of the neck, slightly above the larynx and thyroid. Grab the proximal end of the neck trachea (above the suture) with forceps, and gently pull the thoracic organs (heart, lungs, trachea, and main vessels) *en bloc* from the cavity. Cut the aorta and esophagus at the level of the diaphragm, in order to free the thoracic organs.

Proceed with the removal of the heart, leaving the lungs, larynx, trachea, and thyroid together. To isolate the heart from the lungs, grasp the heart by the blood vessel tree (*see* **Note 5**) and carefully cut the main vessels using scissors. Transfer the organ to the buffered formalin-filled container.

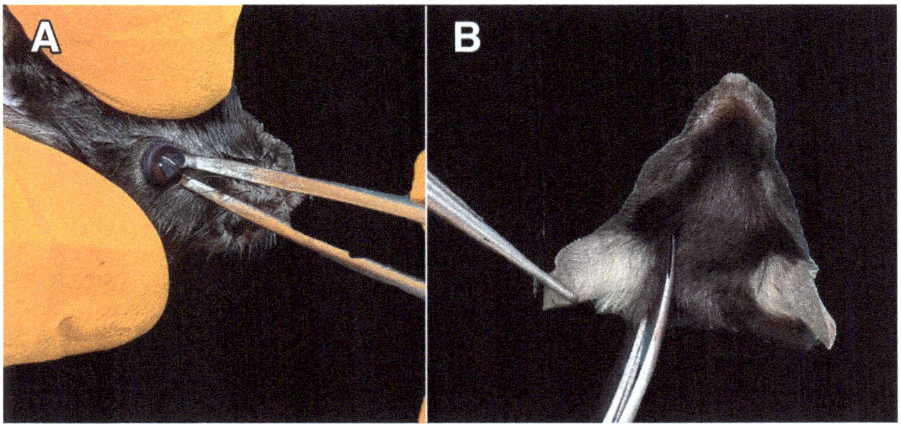

Fig. 12 (**a**) Removing the eye and optic nerve. (**b**) Sampling of the external ear

The thyroid consists of two small lobes adherent to the lateral and dorsal surfaces of the trachea. It is removed and transferred to the buffered formalin-filled container *en bloc*, with the rest of the thoracic organs.

3.6 Head and Cranial Cavity

Each eye is sampled together with the optic nerve and Harderian glands. Remove the eye by inserting a pair of pointed, curved forceps into the orbital cavity, right behind the eye bulb. Gently grab the optic nerve, and isolate the eye by pulling outward and cutting the connective tissue (Fig. 12a). After extirpation, transfer the eye to Davidson's fixative for 24–48 h and then into 90% ethanol for another 24–48 h, and lastly into 4% buffered formalin until processing.

The external ear is removed at the base, cut lengthwise in two halves, and transferred to the formalin-fixed container (Fig. 12b).

The procedure for the opening of the scull and extraction of the brain is shown in Fig. 13.

For the sampling of the spine, place the animal on the dissection board with the dorsal side up. Cut the skin along the midline of the spine. Fold the skin to the left and right side of the animal, exposing the spine. Using large scissors, detach the front limbs from the spine by cutting the scapulae off. Starting from the base of the tail to the neck, cut the pelvic bones and the ribs as close to the spine as possible, on both sides. Lift the tail with forceps, and cut the connective tissue on the ventral side of the spinal column (Fig. 14a). Transfer the removed spinal column to the buffered formalin-filled container, and after 24 h fixation, transfer the sample into a decalcifying solution for 72 h. After 72 h, probe the bone structure using a needle, and if the tissue is soft enough to be cut, make the desired number of samples and submerge them into a calcifying solution for another 48 h before processing.

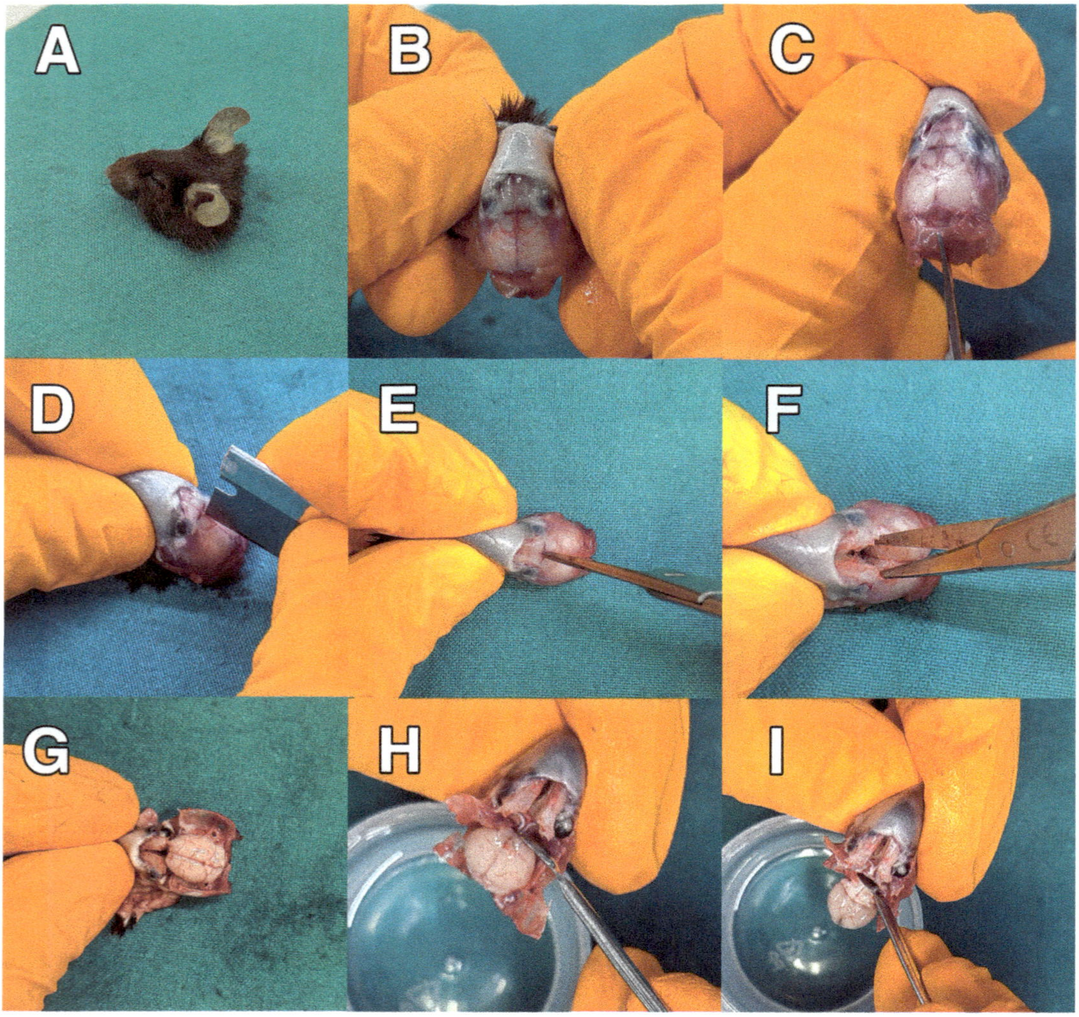

Fig. 13 Cut the cervical spine between the two cervical vertebrae, as close to the base of the scull as possible, using a surgical blade. (**a**) Flip the skin over, exposing the bones of the skull and creating a skin flap that will allow for a better grip during the procedure. (**b**) Insert fine scissors into the spinal cord hole and cut the occipital and intraparietal bones, making sure not to damage the brain tissue (*see* **Note 8**). (**c**) Using a single-edge razor blade, make a shallow incision along the sagittal suture of parietal bones, and another cut along the suture of interparietal and parietal bones. (**d**) Using fine scissors, with their blades oriented along the midline, puncture the frontal bone a little in front of the bregma, making sure not to damage the brain (*see* **Note 9**). (**e**) With the tip of the scissors still inside the newly made puncture, gently rotate the scissors 90° counterclockwise and open them, cracking the calvaria. (**f**) Use blunt forceps to remove fragments of the skull bones and expose the brain. (**g**) Remove the brain by gently pulling it out, using a blunt spatula, and dissecting the optic and cranial nerves along the way. (**h**) Immerse the extirpated brain directly into formalin (**i**) or onto the foil for weighing. (The procedure is adapted from Collins et al. [4])

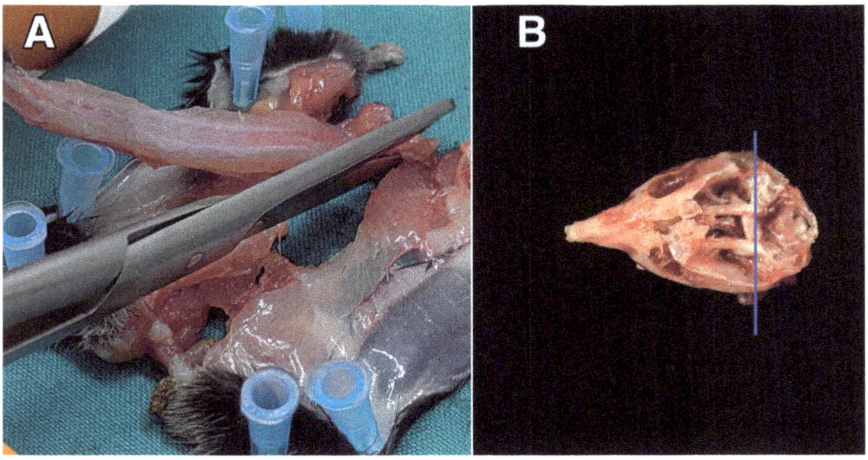

Fig. 14 (**a**) Removal of the spinal cord and (**b**) extraction of the pituitary gland—section line (blue line)

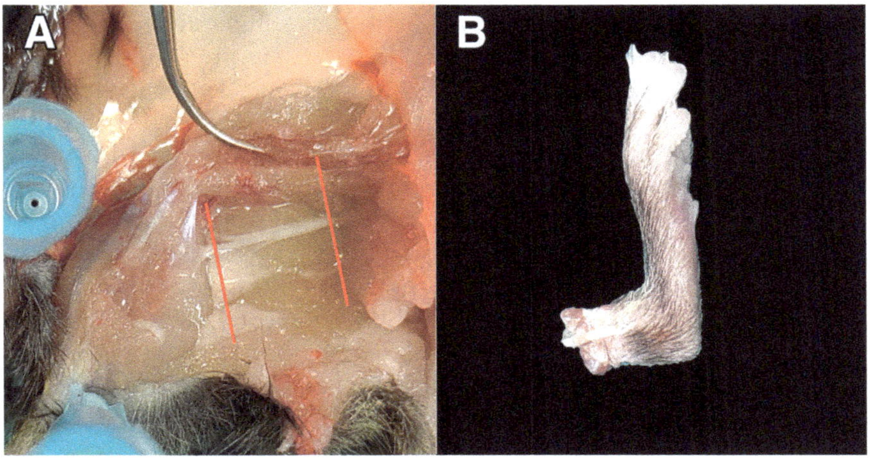

Fig. 15 (**a**) Skeletal muscle and sciatic nerve—section lines of the sciatic nerve (red lines). (**b**) Hind paw

The pituitary gland is located within the *sella turcica* of the sphenoid bone. After extirpation of the brain, it appears as a round gland, covered by a thin membrane (*dura matter*) in the ventral aspect of the skull. The pituitary gland is sampled by cutting through the membrane with a scalpel and removing the gland with round forceps (Fig. 14b).

3.7 Skeletal Muscle, Bones, and Peripheral Nerve

For the sampling of the skeletal muscle and sciatic nerve, dissect and remove the following muscles: *m. gracilis*, *m. adductor*, *m. semimembranosus,* and *m. semitendinosus* from the medial aspect of the thigh (Fig. 15a). Cut the nerve and the underlying muscle at proximal and distal points and transfer them into a container filled with buffered formalin.

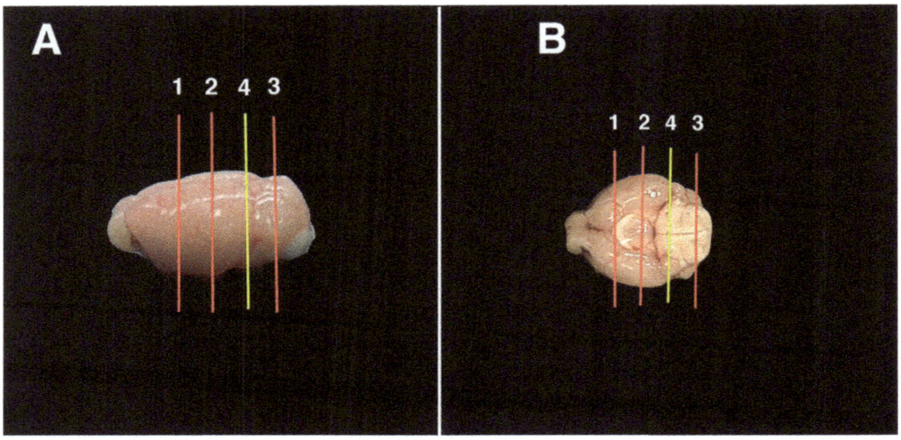

Fig. 16 (**a**) Lateral view of the brain and (**b**) ventral view of the brain (**a** and **b**: 1—level of the optical chiasm, 2—level of the hippocampus, 3—level of pons, 4—level of cerebellum and medulla oblongata)

For the examination of the changes in the skeletal system, the paws are cut with large scissors slightly above the ankle and are transferred to the buffered formalin-filled container (Fig. 15b).

3.8 Sampling of the Organs for Histopathological Analysis

After fixation, the brain is sampled together with the cerebellum and brain stem. In order to minimize the damage to the sensitive brain tissue, special care is required when handling the brain tissue.

Three sections of the brain are routinely embedded (Fig. 16a, b): (1) The first section is made at the level of the optical chiasm and includes the cortex, septum, basal ganglia, and anterior hypothalamus. (2) The second section is made at the level of the hippocampus and it includes the cortex and brain stem at the diencephalon–mesencephalic transition. (3) The third section contains the cerebellum and medulla oblongata. The fourth section is recommended when the investigation of the pons is required.

In order to achieve consistent, precise cuts at the exact same levels of the brain, matrix molds, appropriate for the brain size, can be used (Fig. 17a).

The eye is sampled to ensure that the optic nerve is in the section plane, together with the anterior eye chamber, ocular lens, and Harderian gland (Fig. 17b).

For inhalation toxicology studies, samples from the nasal cavity can be made after the decalcification of the entire scull. Structures of the teeth and palate are used for orientation, in order to make transverse sections of the nasal cavity at consistent levels, since recognition of degenerative and proliferative lesions of various epithelial cell types of the nasal cavity and paranasal sinuses, requires several sections at different levels. In mice, three levels should be examined in inhalation toxicity studies. In oral toxicity studies, only the third sectioning level needs to be examined [5–8]. The sectioning levels are (Fig. 18a): (1) immediately posterior to the incisors,

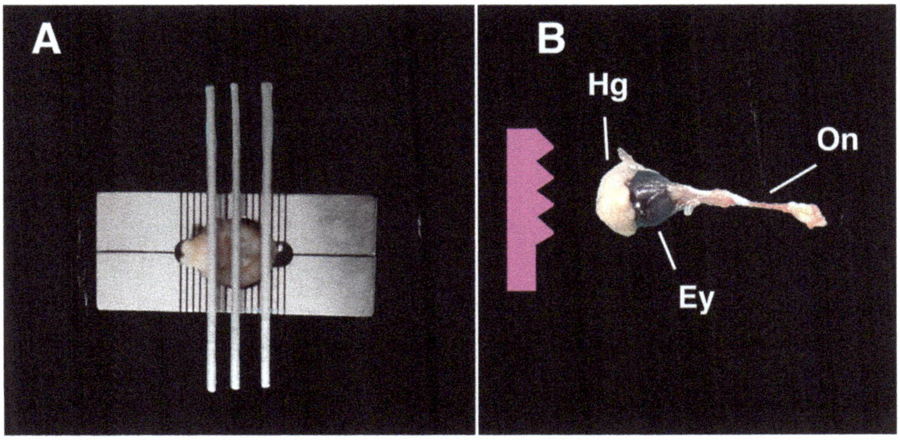

Fig. 17 (**a**) Brain slicer with inserted blades and (**b**) eye (Ey—eye bulb, On—optical nerve, Hg—Harderian gland)

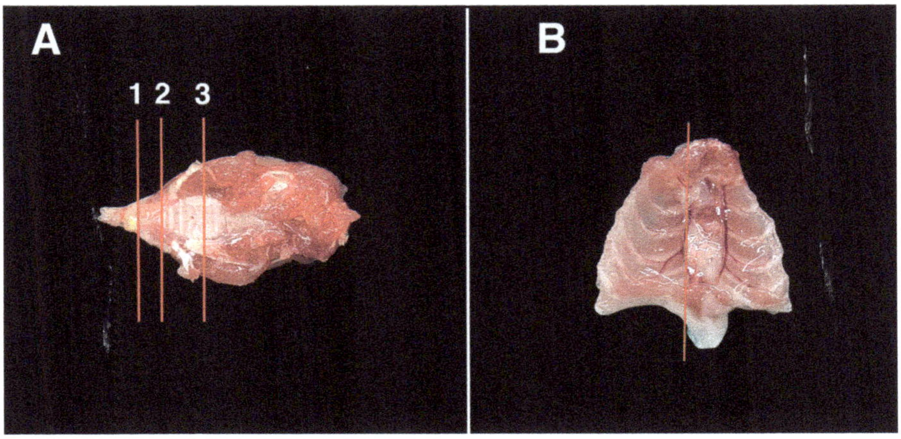

Fig. 18 (**a**) Base of the scull, ventral aspect. (**b**) Sternum

(2) at the level of the incisory papillae, and (3) through the middle of the second molar.

The Zymbal's glands consist of several lobules of modified sebaceous glands, located at the base of the external acoustic meatus. A section through the base of the skull, at the level of the external acoustic meatus, will result in several lobules of gland tissue.

The sternum is transferred into decalcifying solution after 24 h fixation in 10% buffered formalin. After 72 h in decalcifying solution, cut the sample next to the midline, submerge back into decalcifying solution for another 48 h, and process and embed in paraffin on its side (Fig. 18b).

In mice, the thyroid gland consists of two symmetric nodes located on lateral sides, and partially on the dorsal side, of the trachea. Parathyroid glands are located in the vicinity or within

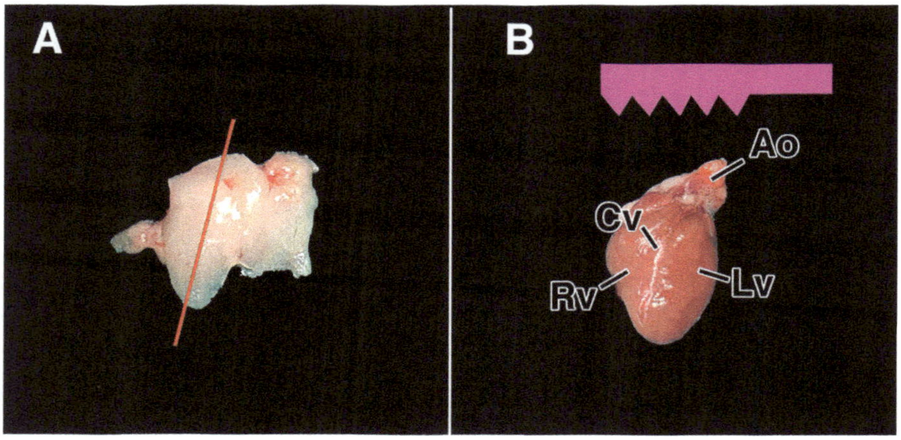

Fig. 19 (**a**) Thymus, section plane. (**b**) Heart, section plane (Rv—right ventricle, Lv—left ventricle, Ao—aorta, Cv—conoventricular vein)

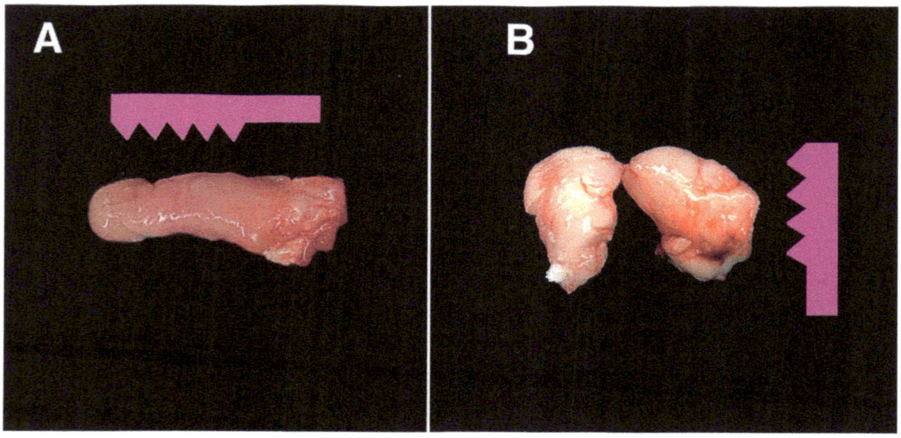

Fig. 20 (**a**) Tongue, lateral aspect and (**b**) salivary glands

the thyroid gland and are not grossly visible. For examination, one transverse section from the esophagus, trachea, thyroid, and parathyroid gland is taken.

The thymus consists of two lobes, is fixed in its entirety, cut, and embedded along one of its lobes (Fig. 19a).

Salivary glands are sampled with a longitudinal cut through the entire length of both glands (Fig. 20b).

The tongue is sampled with a longitudinal section, throughout its entire length (Fig. 20a).

The pharynx and larynx are sampled together in two transversal sections.

For inhalation studies, the trachea is sampled longitudinally in the bifurcation region (carina), since the damage from the inhaled particles is the most prominent in that region (Fig. 21a) [6–8].

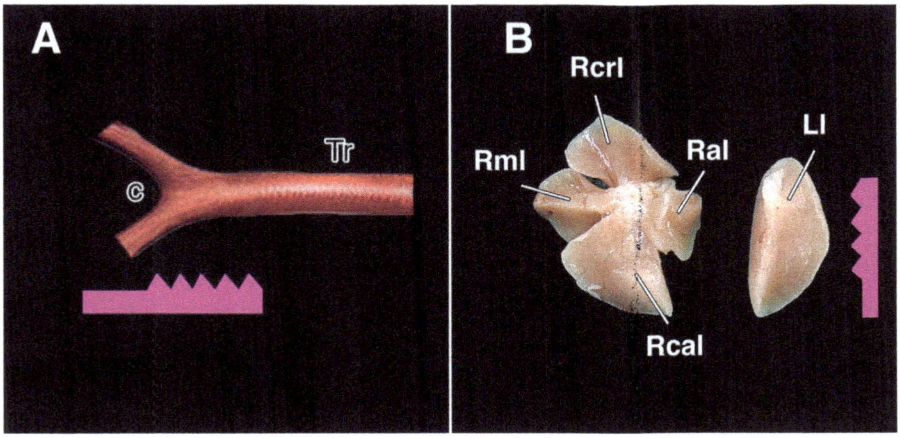

Fig. 21 (**a**) Trachea—graphical presentation (C—carina tracheae, Tr—trachea). (**b**) Lung lobes (Ll—left lung, Rcrl—right cranial lobe, Rml—right medial lobe, Rcal—right caudal lobe, Ral—right accessory lobe)

During the removal of the lungs from the thoracic cavity, the aorta is cut at the level of the diaphragm, and after fixation, a sample is taken from the last 1 cm of its length.

Lungs consist of five lobes: left lobe and right cranial, right medial, right caudal, and right accessory lobe. In inhalation studies, the whole lungs must be sampled according to the scheme (Fig. 21b). The left lung is longitudinally cut, and the right cranial lobe is separated from the rest of the lung. Both sections of the left lung lobe are embedded with the cut surface down. All right lung lobes are embedded with the hilar side down.

For histopathological examination of the heart, a lengthwise cut through both atrium/ventricles should be made, from the base to the apex of the heart (Fig. 19b).

Spleen is sampled in its widest region. Three cross-sections are sampled (Fig. 22a).

The pancreas is made up of two lobes, left and right. The left one is close to the spleen, and the right one is adjacent to the duodenum. One transversal section of each of the lobes is taken for sampling.

The stomach has two distinct regions: the proventricular, or anterior region (Fig. 22b) which is white in color, and the glandular region which is more reddish and has a thicker wall (Fig. 22b). Two regions are demarcated with a limiting ridge (Fig. 22b). Duodenum is located past the stomach, and it contains Brunner's glands in its submucosa. For histological examination, two sections of the gastric mucosa are sampled. First, from the cardiac region of the stomach, across the fundus and antrum up to the duodenal sphincter (Fig. 22b, 1), and second is taken from the forestomach through the fundic area (Fig. 22b, 2). The third sample through the fundic area is optional (Fig. 22b, 3).

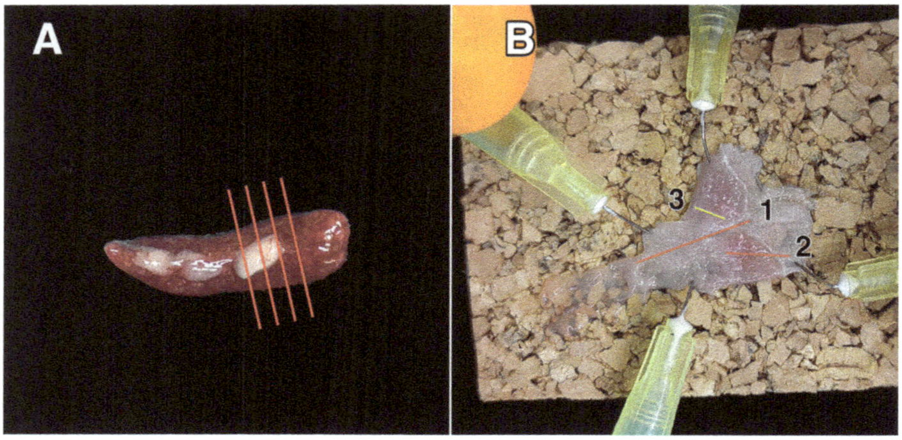

Fig. 22 (**a**) Spleen ventral aspect and (**b**) stomach sampling regions: 1—from antrum to duodenal sphincter, 2—forestomach and fundic area, and 3—fundic area

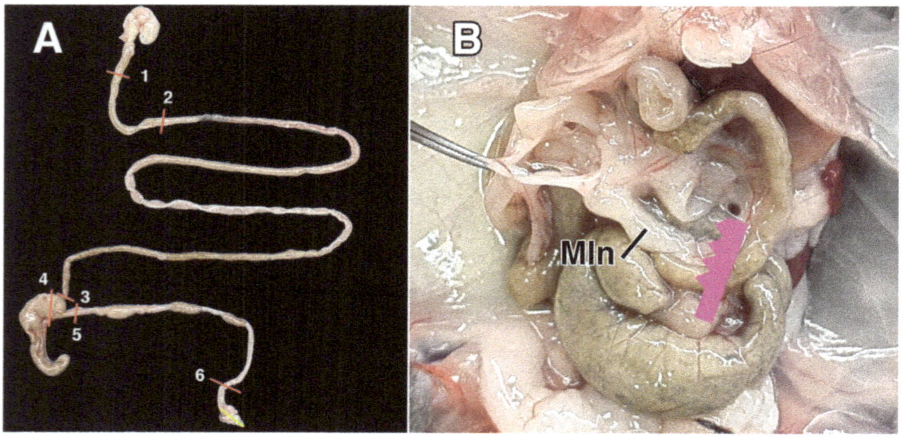

Fig. 23 (**a**) Sampling scheme for the intestine and (**b**) mesenteric lymph nodes (Mln—mesenteric lymph nodes)

Duodenum is sampled 1 cm distal from the pyloric sphincter together with the stomach (Fig. 23a, 1). The next 1 cm of jejunum is sampled at three levels (Fig. 23a, 2). The ileum is sampled 1 cm proximal to the caecum at three levels (Fig. 23a, 3). The caecum is removed, along with a small part of the distal ileum, opened along the greater curvature, and after rinsing with saline solution, placed in 10% buffered formalin. If needed, the caecum is sampled at its greatest diameter (Fig. 23a, 4). Colon is sampled at three levels at its proximal (Fig. 23a, 5) and distal end (Fig. 23a, 6). The rectum is sampled longitudinally in its last 1–2 cm, if it is necessary to include anal muscles in the analysis.

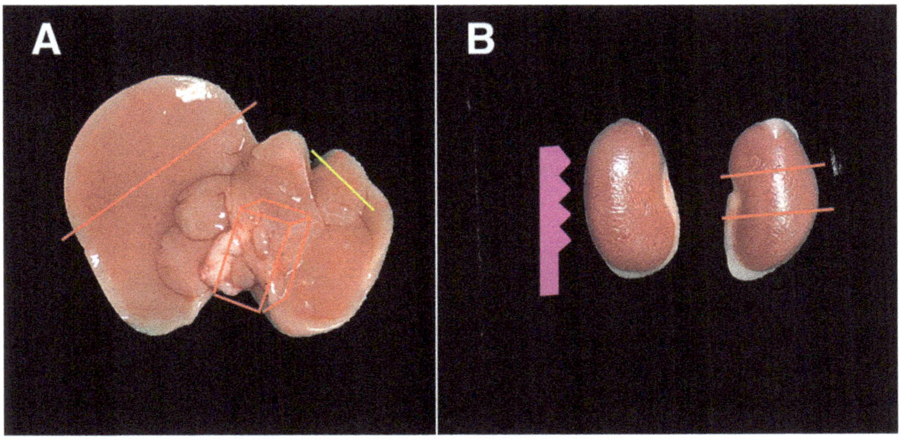

Fig. 24 (**a**) Macroscopic view of the ventral side of the liver—transversal section of the left lateral lobe (red line), longitudinal section of the gallbladder with left and right medial lobes (red box), transversal section through the caudate lobe (yellow line). (**b**) Kidney sampling scheme—section lines (red line)

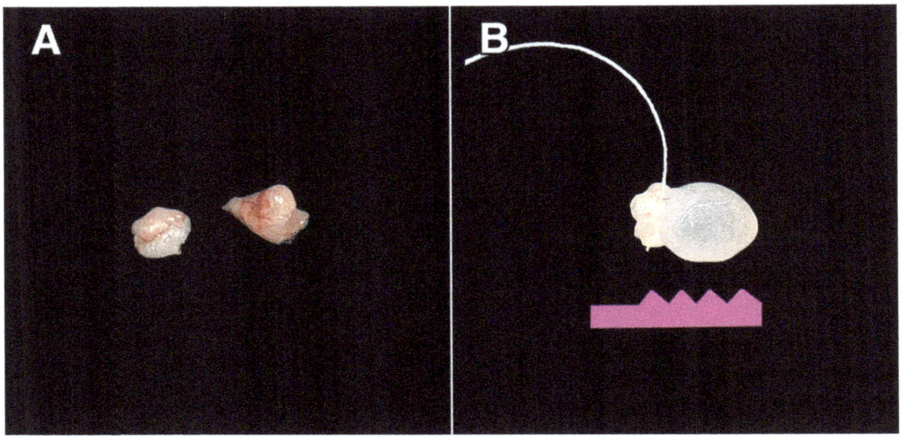

Fig. 25 (**a**) Adrenal glands and (**b**) urinary bladder

Mesenteric lymph nodes are sampled by a longitudinal cut through the mesenteric fat tissue that contains the lymph nodes (Fig. 23b).

For histological examination of the liver, two samples are taken: a transversal section of the left lateral lobe, and a longitudinal section of the gallbladder with left and right medial lobes (Fig. 24a). Optionally, the transversal section through the caudate lobe can be taken.

Both kidneys are sampled for histopathological analysis. The right kidney is cut longitudinally and the left kidney is cut transversely just above or below the hilum (Fig. 24b).

For histopathological evaluation, both adrenal glands are sampled as a whole (Fig. 25a).

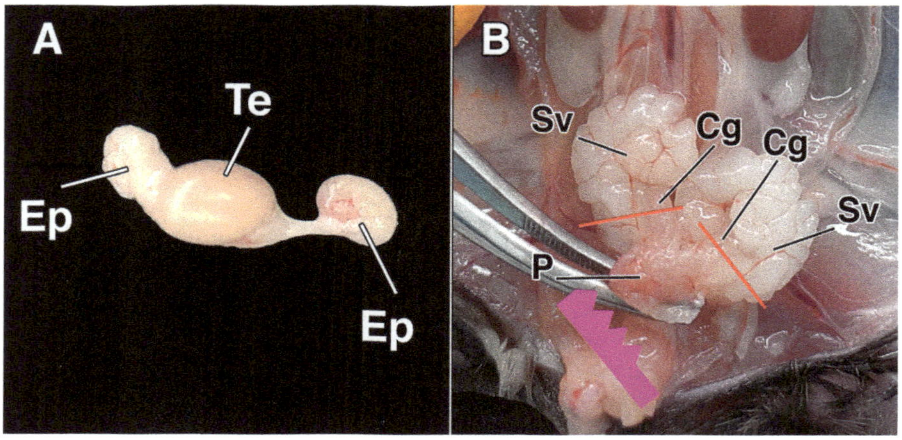

Fig. 26 (**a**) Testis and epididymis (Te—testis, Ep—epididymis). (**b**) Prostate, seminal vesicles, and coagulation gland (P—prostate, Sv—seminal vesicles, Cg—coagulating glands)

The ureter is sampled with the surrounding fat tissue. One transversal cut is sampled.

After fixation, the urinary bladder is cut longitudinally and the ventral portion is sampled (Fig. 25b).

After fixation, for histopathological evaluation, one longitudinal section of each testis and epididymis is made (Fig. 26a).

For histopathological evaluation of the male genital accessory glands, one transversal section through the seminal vesicles and coagulation glands is made. The prostate is cut transversely and sampled as a whole (Fig. 26b).

For histopathological examination of the female genital system, one longitudinal section through each ovary and oviduct is taken. One transversal section through each of the uterine horns, and one longitudinal section through the uterine body, cervix, and vagina are also taken (Fig. 27). Clitoris and vulva are sampled separately.

For the evaluation of skeletal muscle and peripheral nerve, transversal and longitudinal cuts of the *m. biceps femoris* and *n. ischiadicus* are made. A sample is taken by making proximal and distal transverse cuts of the *m. biceps femoris*.

4 Notes

1. When cutting the jugular vein for exsanguination of the animal, be careful not to cut the trachea, since through the opening blood could descend into the lungs.
2. When affixing the animal to the dissection board, make sure that the needle goes through large muscle mass in the extremities and not just the skin.

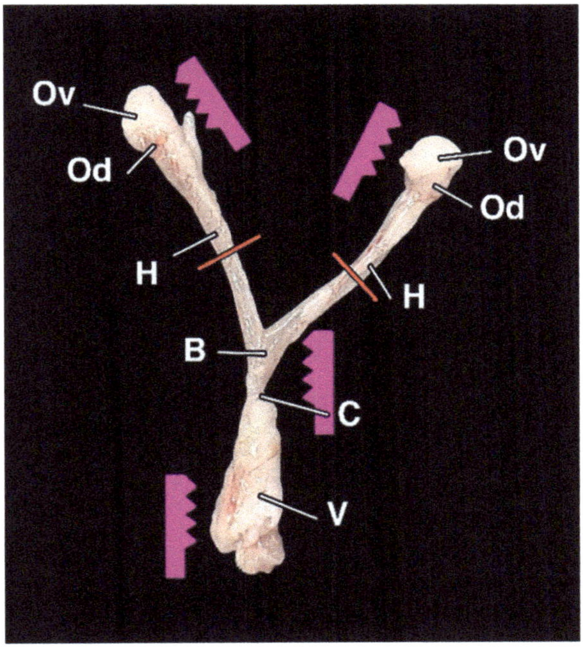

Fig. 27 Uterus with ovaries (Ov—ovary, Od—oviduct, H—uterine horn, B—uterine body, C—uterine cervix, V—vagina)

3. Place the cork-board plate with the skin sample tissue side down in the formalin-filled container, to ensure the tissue is fully submerged and will be properly fixed.
4. Pinch the abdominal wall with blunt forceps and pull it upward to create space between the abdominal wall and abdominal organs, and reduce the probability of accidentally cutting the intra-abdominal organ.
5. Never grasp the organs directly with forceps, since it can damage the tissue.
6. Place the cork-board plate with the stomach sample tissue side down in the formalin-filled container, to ensure the tissue is fully submerged and will be properly fixed.
7. After inserting the needle inside the trachea, grasp tightly with blunt forceps the trachea and the needle within it, to prevent the outflow of formalin.
8. In order to avoid damaging the brain, keep the tip of the scissors pointing straight up, rather than forward.
9. Since the olfactory bulbus is located directly below the bregma, make the puncture hole a few millimeters to the front of it.

References

1. Merriam-Webster.com Dictionary, Merriam-Webster, https://www.merriam-webster.com/dictionary/necropsy. Accessed 15.12.2022
2. Russell WMS, Burch, RL (1959) The principles of humane experimental technique. Methuen: London, UK. https://doi.org/10.5694/j.1326-5377.1960.tb73127.x. Hukkanen RR, Dybdal et al (2019) Scientific and Regulatory Policy Committee points to consider*: the toxicologic pathologist's role in the 3Rs. Toxicol Pathol 47(7), 789–798. https://doi.org/10.1177/0192623319859261
3. Covelli V. Guide to the necropsy of the mouse. http://eulep.pdn.cam.ac.uk/Necropsy_of_the_Mouse/printable.php. Accessed 15.12.2022
4. Collins SC, Wagner C et al (2018) A method for parasagittal sectioning for neuroanatomical quantification of brain structures in the adult mouse. Curr Protocol Mouse Biol 8(3):e48. https://doi.org/10.1002/cpmo.48
5. Ruehl-Fehlert C, Kittel B et al (2003) Revised guides for organ sampling and trimming in rats and mice – Part 1. Exp Toxicol Pathol 55(2–3): 91–106
6. Kittel B, Ruehl-Fehlert et al (2004) Revised guides for organ sampling and trimming in rats and mice – Part 2. A joint publication of the RITA and NACAD groups. Exp Toxicol Pathol 55(6):413–431. https://doi.org/10.1078/0940-2993-00349
7. Morawietz G, Ruehl-Fehlert C et al (2004) Revised guides for organ sampling and trimming in rats and mice – Part 3. A joint publication of the RITA and NACAD groups. Exp Toxicol Pathol 55(6):433–449. https://doi.org/10.1078/0940-2993-00350
8. Fiette L, Slaoui M (2011) Necropsy and sampling procedures in rodents. Methods Mol Biol 691:39–67. https://doi.org/10.1007/978-1-60761-849-2_3

INDEX

Maja Čemažar, Tanja Jesenko and Urša Lampreht Tratar (eds.), *Mouse Models of Cancer: Methods and Protocols*, Methods in Molecular Biology, vol. 2773, https://doi.org/10.1007/978-1-0716-3714-2,

© The Editor(s) (if applicable) and The Author(s), under exclusive license to Springer Science+Business Media, LLC, part of Springer Nature 2024

GPSR Compliance
The European Union's (EU) General Product Safety Regulation (GPSR) is a set of rules that requires consumer products to be safe and our obligations to ensure this.

If you have any concerns about our products, you can contact us on

ProductSafety@springernature.com

In case Publisher is established outside the EU, the EU authorized representative is:

Springer Nature Customer Service Center GmbH
Europaplatz 3
69115 Heidelberg, Germany

www.ingramcontent.com/pod-product-compliance
Ingram Content Group UK Ltd.
Pitfield, Milton Keynes, MK11 3LW, UK
UKHW052005051026
15624UKWH00003B/567
* 9 7 8 1 0 7 1 6 3 7 1 3 5 *